CONFRONT CANCER

CONFRONT CANCER

Tools to Make the Right Decisions for Your Cancer

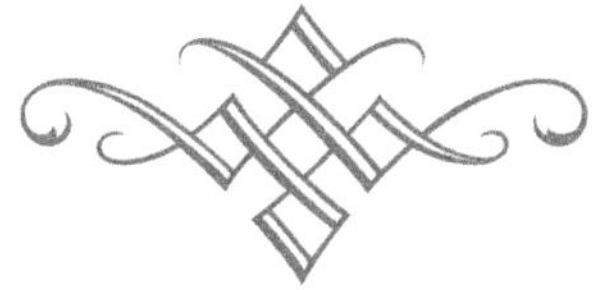

JOSIE HAYES, PhD

Waltham, Massachusetts
2022

ISBN hardback: 979-8-9857019-0-6
paperback: 979-8-9857019-3-7

Book and Cover design by: Tamian Wood, BeyondDesignBooks.com

This book is not intended as a substitute for the medical advice of physicians.

CONTENTS

Prologue ix

Ch. 1. Why Read This Book? 1

Ch. 2. What Is Cancer? 11

How Cancer Begins 11

How Is Cancer Classified? 14

Anatomical Site, Subtypes, and Stages 15

Skin Cancer as an Example 17

Who Comes Up with the Guidelines for Clinical Diagnosis? 21

Metastasis and Its Relevance to Diagnosis and Staging 13

Ch.3. Diagnosing Cancer 27

Tumor Imaging 27

Tumor Biopsy 32

Ch.4. Genetic Tests and Samples 41

Genetic Tests for Tumors 43

Circulating Tumor DNA 43

Germline Genetic Testing 46

Considerations for Genetic Testing 48

Ch. 5. Understanding Your Test Results 53

Laboratory Reports 56

Failed Tests 57

Getting a Second Opinion....................................58
Ch. 6. Cancer Therapy..61
Types of Therapy..61
Traditional Therapies...61
Targeted Therapies...62
Ch. 7. Using Your Diagnostic Information to Inform Treatment Options..73
Clinical Trials 76
Statistics Associated with Your Treatment 93
Decision-Making Checklist for Treatment 95
Ch. 8. Forming a Plan 103
Take Time to Process 104
Research Your Health Care Team 105
Formulate a Testing and Treatment Plan 109
Consider a Second Opinion.................................112
Make a Decision That's Right for You...............114
Prepare for Your Treatment..................................116
Ch. 9. What If the Cancer Returns?...............................119
Ch. 10. Conclusion 125
Helpful Organizations & Useful Links..........................129
Glossary & Cancer Terminology....................................133
Bibliography & Further Reading.....................................139

PROLOGUE

Having worked in cancer for over fifteen years, I find that my friends and family members have often called upon me when they learn they have the "Big C." I have been able to help them discuss test results with their doctor and navigate treatment options. In every case, I assisted the person and their family in understanding their diagnosis and how to use it to have the best outcome from their treatment. I wrote this book to provide the same advice to you and to help you find the information you need to make an informed decision about your treatment.

The first experience I had working with cancer was as a clinical scientist at a hospital in Leeds, United Kingdom. During this time, I learned to diagnose cancers by looking at their genetic makeup under the microscope—a subject called *cytogenetics.* However, over the ten years I worked there, I noticed the method of diagnosing some cancer types didn't change. So, I decided to leave my post at the hospital to do a PhD in brain cancer, hoping I could help to change that. Following my PhD, I worked for another three years on the academic study of brain cancer, which took me across the Atlantic to San Francisco. I looked at brain tumors using deep, digitized genetic methods called next-generation sequencing. Eventually, I moved to work in the biotechnology industry in Silicon Valley at a company that develops therapeutics to treat cancer. In this role, I identify features of cancer to predict whether a patient will respond to a particular treatment.

This book is for newly diagnosed cancer patients or patients who have been presented with new options for treatment, and their families and friends. The complicated information given to a patient can be daunting, and it comes at a very difficult time in the patient's life. This book is designed to help clarify the complex information the doctor puts forward and dig even deeper into which are the optimal tests to have done and how to navigate the results to ensure the best treatment options.

I organized this book into nine chapters, which you can read in any order. However, I recommend that you first read through Chapters 1 and 2 to get a general understanding of what cancer is. Then the other sections will provide the necessary background and resources to inform you along your decision-making journey. Finally, in Chapter 8, we will go through the steps to arrive at a plan for the cancer treatment that is right for you.

Throughout the book, I refer to particular clinical and scientific studies that have been carried out; these are listed in the reference section at the end of the book so that you can find out more about them.

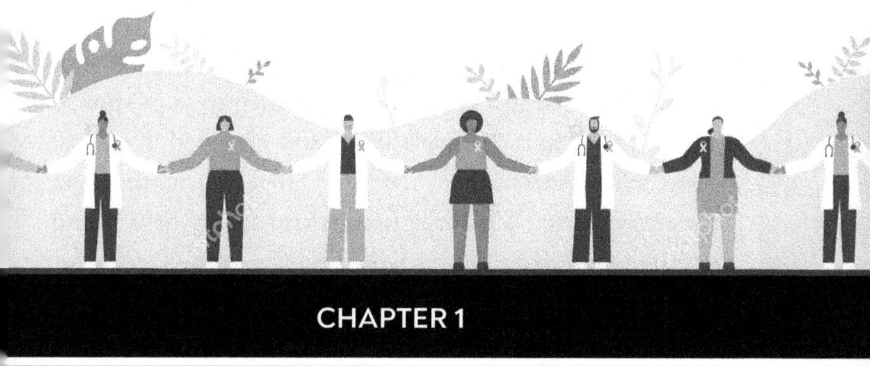

CHAPTER 1

WHY READ THIS BOOK?

Have you ever spoken to someone who has cancer but doesn't know the type of cancer they have? This is not an uncommon scenario. In the 2011 movie *50/50,* Adam Lerner finds out he has schwannoma neurofibrosarcoma after going to the doctor with pain in his back. Once the doctor tells him the diagnosis, he doesn't listen to anything more the doctor says. He comes out of the doctor's office and cannot even pronounce the name of his cancer.

Finding out you have cancer is a huge deal, and processing that information can take time. So, after being informed of a cancer diagnosis, it's no wonder we zone out when the doctor launches into a detailed explanation, often accompanied by a lot of technical jargon.

You may have already experienced the dreaded moment in the doctor's office when you found out you had cancer.

The question is, where do you go from there? You are suddenly immersed in a world that feels alien to you—poked and prodded in a clinician's office and included in discussions where there are so many technical terms that you are entirely lost. When my friends and family have found themselves in that exact situation, they've turned to me for help. I am not a medical doctor, but I have spent almost two decades diagnosing cancer in labs in the hospital and studying it at top-tier research institutions. I wrote this book to help more people navigate this challenging time in their lives.

There are hundreds of types of cancers. The Big C can arise anywhere in the body, and a tumor in one person may differ greatly from one in the same location in another person. We can detect the differences by looking at pieces of the tumor under the microscope or performing tests to see which genetic alterations the tumor harbors. Scientists in the laboratory define features of the tumor and doctors perform scans of your body, which allows your health care team to characterize your tumor as a type of cancer.

In society, we are used to defining cancer by the body part where the cancer is found, but this is a somewhat oversimplified view of a cancer diagnosis. For example, when a doctor observes several tumors in different organs of a patient, which organ should be used for the diagnosis? If one person's cancer type differs from another but they are both in the lung, how is this difference reflected in the diagnosis? By looking at patterns of cancer under the microscope and testing their genetics, scientists can assign tumors into predefined bins that researchers and doctors have put together based on their collective learning during cancer research. The bin to which your tumor is assigned is your diagnosis, which is the term I will use in the rest of the book. Because your treatment plan is based on your diagnosis, it is essential you get the right diagnosis.

Doctors know how people with a specific cancer diagnosis generally respond when they receive certain treatments. Your health care team can provide you with this "performance" information, along with other information about you that may influence your experience with a specific treatment, so you can devise a treatment plan. As a simple example, your cancer diagnosis may suggest that there are three viable options for treatment. The data indicate that patients with your diagnosis respond to all three treatments similarly. However, one of these treatments may interfere with another medication you take, while another has side effects that you are not willing to tolerate. Only one treatment remains as a best option for you.

*Because your treatment plan is based on your diagnosis, **it is essential you get the right diagnosis.***

New cancer treatments are coming out all the time. These improve upon previous treatments in how effective they are, their ease of administration (e.g., oral rather than intravenous), and their lower rates of severe side effects. Frequently, though, the testing tools needed to identify patients who are suitable for these drugs lag significantly behind the drugs' availability.

For example, genetic alterations in a protein called EGFR (epidermal growth factor receptor) were first reported in lung cancers in the early 2000s, and this discovery was quickly followed by clinical trials showing that patients with tumors harboring an EGFR alteration were sensitive to drugs that target the EGFR protein (EGFR inhibitors). However, it was not until seven years later that regulatory bodies issued the first provisional recommendation to routinely test lung cancers for alterations in the EGFR protein. Therefore, for seven years, doctors did not know whether their patients should take the drug even though it was available.

Several years on, despite the continued availability of EGFR inhibitors, not all patients are tested for EGFR alterations. In 2019, community hospitals tested only 54 percent of patients with lung cancer for an EGFR alteration. That means that out of one hundred patients with lung cancer, only fifty-four took a test to allow them to

> *That means that out of one hundred patients with lung cancer, only fifty-four took a test to allow them to receive the optimal drug for their disease.*

receive the optimal drug for their disease. The EGFR mutation is the most frequently tested genetic alteration in lung cancer, which means there is even less testing for patients with tumors harboring other genetic alterations.

There are several reasons for this lack of testing, many of them due to logistics that can undoubtedly be improved by better management of diagnosis efforts. Health care professionals expressed their dissatisfaction with the current state of molecular testing in a 2020 questionnaire. Despite their concerns, only half of the health care community stated their agency had a policy or strategy in place to address these concerns. You can improve the odds for yourself by getting the right doctor and being proactive about the testing strategy they use.

In most cases, your cancer diagnosis will be reasonably straightforward; the different tests you have will all point to the same answer, and your doctor will have an effortless time providing you with a diagnosis. However, in some cases, the picture may not be quite so clear. Some tests may show ambiguous results, and different tests may even suggest a different diagnosis. In this event, it is much more difficult for a doctor and health care team to come to a conclusion. But your doctor will let you know if you have a scenario like this, and testing laboratories will write this in the reports you receive from them.

Misdiagnosis is a genuine problem, and it happens for many reasons. Examples are inadequate quality biopsies, human error, or a cancer that just does not fit into one of the known diagnoses. This scenario is often obvious during the diagnostic journey, but sometimes you and your doctor can believe you have a precise diagnosis when that is not the case. It is possible that in this scenario you may never find out your health care team misdiagnosed you.

Computer-aided diagnosis sheds even more light on the matter. Google trains its advanced artificial intelligence models to diagnose cancers. In these models, the computer learns by being given two pieces of information: cancer testing results and the diagnosis given by doctors. After training the computer, it can diagnose other cancers when given data with an unknown diagnosis. In one study comparing the computer diagnosis to the human diagnosis, the computer achieved an absolute reduction of 5.7 percent in **false positives** and 9.4 percent in **false negatives**.

The potential effects of this are huge. At the population level, a large percentage of patients are not getting the best treatment available for their cancer. At the individual level, misdiagnosis will lead to an ineffective treatment, and hence the tumor will continue to grow. The treatment given may have side effects that are undesirable or cause lasting damage, which could have been avoided with the right diagnosis. You may eventually have another **biopsy** and receive a new, correct diagnosis and treatment plan, but only after suffering unnecessarily.

To repeat, your treatment plan is based on your diagnosis: **it is essential you get the right diagnosis**.

A Mayo clinic study in 2017 reported that the referral diagnosis and final diagnosis were distinctly different in 21 percent of cases, highlighting the difficulties in reaching the appropriate diagnosis, and illustrating that not every institution has the expertise or resources to make a concrete diagnosis. It also shows that getting a second opinion is extremely valuable.

Misdiagnosis is such a problem that countless legal experts specialize in this exact area. A quick Google search for "cancer misdiagnosis" shows many hits from law firms offering their services to patients who have experienced this.

Knowing all of this, or having experienced it, can make you suspicious of your doctor or your health care team, but that shouldn't be so. Your doctor is highly trained, very knowledgeable, and on your side. The point of you arming yourself with this knowledge is so that you can be a part of the team taking care of you. Do your research and show it to your doctor. Record your meetings or take notes when you meet with your doctor so you can go back to what was said as questions arise in your mind.

This is your body, and these are ultimately your decisions.

This is your life.

You want to make sure you have the best advice from the best health care team, which will provide you with an excellent base of data to make informed decisions about your treatment.

Although we put cancer into bins for ease of diagnosis, everyone's cancer is unique. Your tumor may be in the same organ of the body as someone else's, and it may even look similar under the microscope. However, the genetic alterations in your tumor are not likely to be the same as anyone else's. During the past decade, cancer management plans have been increasingly designed to provide personalized treatment options for a patient, an approach known as **personalized medicine**. These strategies mean that even if your neighbor has the same type of cancer as you, you may have different treatment options offered to you. You can work this to your advantage by finding out as much as you can about your cancer, which will open more doors for personalized therapy. It will not only improve your outcome but could also help you avoid treatments with terrible side effects.

Making informed decisions on your treatment requires having as much accurate information on **your unique cancer** as you can. You can then look up information about how others with a similar type of cancer did on a specific treatment. This is usually available as statistical information, and we will discuss this further in Chapter 7.

Hopefully, you are beginning to see that a cancer diagnosis is very complex, and it is the cornerstone of your treatment plan. Over the next few chapters, I hope to convince you just how intricate cancer is, and help you understand the challenges that lie behind every aspect of the investigation of your tumor. With this knowledge, you will be able to discuss which tests you are having—and the implications of their results—with your doctor. You will learn how to seek the best second opinion possible, and how to put together the information you obtain from both doctors to formulate a treatment plan with your health care team that is right for **you**.

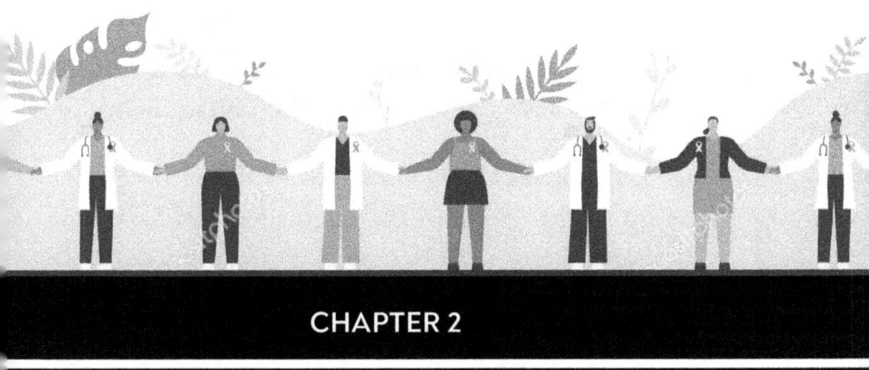

CHAPTER 2

WHAT IS CANCER?

HOW CANCER BEGINS

Cancer begins in one of the fundamental building blocks of the human body: the cell. A cell is about a tenth of a millimeter in size and consists mainly of a colorless, gel-like substance surrounded by a membrane. We have around thirty trillion cells in our body, of many different types, all working together to form our organs. But many of these cells do not form a fixed population; there is a constant turnover, with some cells dying and new ones taking their place. Within the cell is a nucleus that houses your genetic material. As your cells are dividing and renewing themselves, this genetic material—DNA—needs to reproduce itself in order to spread to the new generation of cells. This process of DNA copying and reproduction is called **replication**. Sometimes things go wrong in replicating the genetic material within the nucleus, causing genetic alterations (**mutations**).

Each cell's nucleus contains a copy of the entire genetic makeup of that person—the instructions for how each cell should behave. Under normal circumstances, cells are under tight regulation, so they grow and divide when needed in response to specific cues provided by other cells. When a cell becomes old or damaged, it dies (a process called **apoptosis**). In cancer, the cells escape this tight regulation, grow uncontrollably, and spread into the surrounding tissues.

Most cancers begin in tissue cells and take the form of a solid mass, known as a tumor. This process can occur in any cell; for example, a bone cell, muscle cell, or fat cell. Cancer may also develop from a blood-producing cell in the bone marrow. This is called *leukemia*.

Cancer refers specifically to the growth of cells that infiltrate the surrounding tissues; these are **malignant** tumors. If an overgrowth of cells occurs but does not invade the surrounding tissues, this is a **benign** tumor and not cancer. Benign tumors are usually not threatening unless they arise in the brain.

So how does a cell become deviant, escape the usual regulation, and grow uncontrollably? A genetic alteration occurs that provides the cell with an advantage. For example, a cell with a genetic alteration may be able to hide any genetic damage from the usual protection mechanisms, thus escaping death.

Genetic replication is an error-prone process, so our cells have developed sophisticated mechanisms to identify any DNA damage and fix it. Sometimes, though, damage slips through the net, and genetic alterations arise in a cell. These alterations will be passed to any cells that are derived from the original cell, like copies from a Xerox. And DNA replication occurs billions of times every minute in our body—so it stands to reason that as we get older, our cells accumulate more and more of these genetic alterations. Most of these mutations do not affect us, but some of them can cause cancer. Exposure to specific environmental agents, such as smoking and ultraviolet light, can increase the rate at which these genetic alterations arise. That's why exposing your skin to the sun or your lungs to tobacco smoke can cause an increased risk of specific types of cancer.

Cancer cells can also influence the normal cells surrounding them, inducing those cells to support and feed the tumor. For example, cancer cells can emit chemicals that break down the surrounding **microenvironment** to enable the cell to move through it. Cancer cells can also induce the formation of blood vessels around the tumor, which supply oxygen and nutrients to enable it to grow efficiently.

An essential finding of the past twenty years is that cancer can evade the immune system. This is important because our immune system not only guards the body against infection, but it can also protect against the development of cancer. If our immune system detects a genetically changed cell, it will set a process in place to kill that cell. By avoiding the immune system, a cancer cell can escape this surveillance and reproduce uncontrollably.

HOW IS CANCER CLASSIFIED?

The first piece of information you will likely have about your cancer is where it is in your body; this may or may not be the site where the cancer originated. For example, cancer of the colon (or colon cancer) starts in the cells of the colon, and brain cancer starts in the cells of the brain. The tissue or organ in which the tumor initially formed will influence your eventual outcomes and some of your treatment options. While they grow faster than the surrounding normal cells, some cancer cells grow relatively slowly and spread less frequently. Other cancers grow at an extreme rate. In certain parts of the body, such as in the pancreas, it is challenging to detect tumors, and it may be the case that you have had cancer for an extended time before a diagnosis is made.

We can further define cancer by the type of cell in which the initial genetic alteration occurred. Some cancers arise in the cells that cover the surface of the body or organs, called **epithelial cells**. These appear as long fence-like shapes when viewed under a microscope. Certain types of these cells produce mucus, and cancers arising within them are called *adenocarcinomas.* Most cancers of the lung, colon, and prostate are adenocarcinomas. Cells just below the outer surface of organs look flat, like fish scales, under a microscope and are called **squamous cells**. Squamous cells line organs such as the stomach, lungs, and kidneys. Cancer that arises in one of these cells is called *squamous cell carcinoma*.

The genetic changes in every person's cancer are unique. While some cancers in certain parts of the body arise due to genetic alteration, further alterations accumulate throughout the life of the tumor. A genetically unique tumor develops, and some of the genetic changes within that tumor are more critical for treatment than others. It is a huge challenge for science to determine what those mutations are and to develop therapies to target them. There's more information about these new targeted therapies in Chapter 6.

The genetic changes in every person's cancer are unique.

ANATOMICAL SITE, SUBTYPES, AND STAGES

Everyone's cancer is unique, but specific genetic alterations or tumor characteristics seen under the microscope allow us to group cancers into categories (the bins I mentioned earlier). This enables doctors to define treatment plans for groups of tumors that have similar characteristics.

For example, let's suppose you have a diagnosis of lung cancer. This diagnosis opens up your options to a suite of drugs specifically approved for lung cancer, including chemotherapies, targeted inhibitors, and immunotherapy. The specific treatment you get is further refined by how your cancer looks under the microscope: Is mucin present, as in an adenocarcinoma? Do the cells look flat, like those of a squamous cell carcinoma? Then the treatment options can be further refined by the genetic alterations present in the tumor. For example, an alteration in the gene EGFR opens up the possibility of using an EGFR inhibitor to treat the tumor. This information—the way your cancer cells look and what genetic alterations they have—allows doctors to identify the subtype of disease you have.

Usually, your cancer's site of origin will be the site where you were having symptoms. For example, a scan for digestive symptoms may show a tumor in the colon. It is not always as simple as that, however. If you have advanced cancer, it is possible some pieces of the tumor got into your bloodstream and attached to other parts of your body. A body scan might then show tumors at both the **primary** site and at one or more **secondary** sites. Using the characteristics of the cancer cells seen under the microscope and the genetic alterations, it is usually possible to determine the primary cancer site. However, this is not always possible to know, and these cancers are called *cancers of unknown primary.*

So, to recap, the pieces of information needed to diagnose your cancer are the pathology report (how the cancer cells look under the microscope), the genetic report (which DNA mutations your cancer has), and the scan information (where the tumor is in your body). But in addition to knowing your cancer's original site, it is also vital to know its **stage**. The World Health Organization (WHO) defines the stage for each cancer type based on the primary organ it arose in. The extent to which the tumor has infiltrated into surrounding tissues defines the stage, as well as its spread to other parts of the body and its growth rate. Treatments for low-stage cancer are typically less aggressive than those recommended for high-stage cancer.

SKIN CANCER AS AN EXAMPLE

Skin cancer is the most common cancer in the United States, so let's use it as an example for how a diagnosis is reached. Skin cancer is an abnormal growth of skin cells that infiltrate into the surrounding skin. It can begin in any layer of the skin, but most often develops on the outer skin surface, the part that's exposed to ultraviolet light from the sun. The three types of skin cancer are basal cell carcinoma, squamous cell carcinoma, and melanoma.

Basal cell carcinoma usually occurs in the parts of the skin that are most highly exposed to the sun, such as your neck, face, or ears. This type of cancer may appear on the skin as a pearly or waxy bump. It could also look like a flat, brown scar. The second type of skin cancer, squamous cell carcinoma, also occurs in exposed areas of your body. People with darker skin are more likely to develop squamous cell carcinoma in regions that the sun does not reach. This type of tumor appears as a firm, red nodule or a flat lesion with a scaly, crusted surface. And finally, the third most common skin cancer is melanoma, which can occur on any part of your body. However, it most often appears on the face or torso in men and on the lower legs of women. It can affect people of any skin tone. Melanoma appears as a dark brown spot with darker speckles or as a mole that has changed color and may bleed.

The skin layer in which the tumor originally arose provides the basis for classifying and naming these skin cancers. Squamous cell carcinoma originates in the thin, flat squamous cells that form the top layer of the outer skin. Basal cell carcinoma forms in a basal cell, which are round cells that lie just under the squamous cells. Melanoma forms in melanocytes—the cells that make melanin, the pigment that colors our skin.

If you have a suspected skin cancer diagnosis, the doctor will take a sample of cells from the site to test in the laboratory. The doctor may perform any number of standard biopsy procedures to collect the sample; these are discussed in detail in Chapter 3. The piece is tested to determine whether the tissue is cancerous, and to determine the stage of cancer, if needed. There are five stages of basal cell carcinoma and squamous cell carcinoma, which are defined by tumor size and the extent of spread to other regions of the body. Stage 0 is called *carcinoma in situ* (*in situ* is Latin for "situated in the original place") and is the least aggressive type. It refers to abnormal cells that have not moved from their original location and are not considered malignant. In stage I, the cells have grown to a small tumor of two centimeters or smaller. In stage II, the tumor is between two and four centimeters. A tumor must have one of the following three characteristics to be classified as stage III: smaller than four centimeters and spread to one lymph node; larger than four centimeters; or spread below the skin or into the bone. Stage IV skin cancer, the most aggressive form, is diagnosed when it has spread to more than one location (like a lymph node, bone, or other organ).

The example of skin cancer illustrates how the description of your cancer is derived. Your doctor follows guidelines to define which type and stage of cancer you have based on measurable characteristics of your tumor.

The treatments you will be offered will hinge upon this diagnosis and description, and therefore, they must be correct. To add to the diagnosis, information on how aggressive your tumor is or the likelihood of it returning after surgery is also essential.

Let's return to the skin cancer example. In most cases, simple surgery will be effective and complete removal of the tumor can be achieved. During tumor removal, a rim of normal tissue around the edge, termed the **margin**, is also removed. They then analyze the margin tissue to see whether any cancer cells are present. If the margin is defined as *clear or negative,* it means cancer cells have not been detected in this margin tissue, and usually no more surgery is required. If cancer cells are present in the margin tissue, margins are defined as *positive,* and more surgery is typically needed to remove any remaining cancer cells. If the margins are defined as *close,* cancer cells are close to the margin, but not right at the edge.

Your doctor will determine whether there is a low or high risk for the cancer coming back based on

- the margin information
- where in the body the tumor was found
- whether the borders of the lesion were well defined
- whether you have had skin cancer before
- whether the cells have aggressive characteristics under the microscope
- how close it is to nerves

The perception of risk that the doctor gets from this information determines the treatment protocol they will follow. For example, if you have a low-risk basal cell skin cancer with negative margins, you will usually not require more treatment, but will just come in for regular follow-up visits to confirm it has not returned. If you have a high-risk basal cell skin cancer with negative margins but extensive involvement of nerves, the doctor may consider radiotherapy for the tumor site. There's more about radiotherapy in Chapter 6.

WHO COMES UP WITH THE GUIDELINES FOR CLINICAL DIAGNOSIS?

To come up with a consensus classification for diagnosis, the WHO brings together key leaders in the field to determine appropriate subtypes for each cancer. The results of these discussions are available in peer-reviewed papers and the WHO books, which are updated regularly. For example, the most recent update for lung cancer was *The 2015 World Health Organization Classification of Lung Tumors.* This book includes broad separation of lung cancer into epithelial tumors, mesenchymal tumors, lymphohistiocytic tumors, tumors of ectopic origin, and metastatic tumors (tumors that have spread to the lung from another site). They separate each of these five broad types into subtypes. For example, lung cancer epithelial tumors have ten distinct subtypes—and if we look at just one of those subtypes, lung adenocarcinoma, it is further separated into eleven more defined subtypes. So you can see these guidelines are very detailed and specific. The guidelines may look intimidating, but you just need to know the subtypes that refer to your cancer, and most likely only one or two of them will apply.

The very first classification of lung tumors occurred in 1967. The most recent update to these classifications added advances in genetic research and staining techniques for looking at lung cancer cells under the microscope. The arrival of new cancer drugs on the market can also influence these guidelines, as they can dramatically improve the outcome and quality of life for specific groups of patients.

This situation is especially true for targeted therapies, where the drug performs best in a specific group of patients defined by a particular characteristic. For example, patients with lung cancer diagnosed as lung adenocarcinoma with an EGFR mutation will likely have the best outcomes when treated with an EGFR inhibitor.

Metastasis and Its Relevance to Diagnosis and Staging

So far, we have discussed the diagnosis of a tumor situated where it first arose: the primary tumor. But once a cancerous tumor has become established at its primary location, it often infiltrates the surrounding normal tissues. From there, cells can break off from the tumor and go into the body's circulatory system, allowing them to move around the body. In most cases, these cells will die before they can colonize another site, but sometimes they take hold elsewhere and begin to divide. Once a tumor has formed, it will start to make blood vessels. The spreading of cancer to another site is called **metastasis,** and in some cases, it can occur before you have even been diagnosed with cancer. Usually, if metastasis happens before your diagnosis and the new tumors can be seen on your scan, you will be diagnosed with stage IV cancer.

For each cancer type, there are common sites that the tumor may migrate to, which is most likely due to their proximity to the original tumor and well-trodden paths in the circulatory system. For example, lung cancer may colonize another lung lobe or move to the brain, liver, or bones. Colon cancer commonly migrates to the liver and lungs. Breast cancer most often spreads to the bone, brain, liver, or lungs.

The tumor cells at these distant sites still resemble those at the original location. However, there can be some crucial differences because cancer cells can evolve as they grow. Let's look briefly at what that means.

A cancer cell may have limited resources during its lifetime. These may include a lack of space and a lack of nutrients or oxygen. The cancer cells that survive are those that adapt to this restricted environment. The adapted cancer cells may have different genetic alterations than those that die off—alterations that allow them to survive. This means that over time, the proportion of cancer cells adapted to the environment increases in the tumor—a process called evolution—and the genetic composition of the tumor may change. The cancer cells that left the original tumor and colonized another site may have had a particular genetic alteration that conferred their ability to colonize elsewhere. Because the cells at the site of metastasis are descendants of

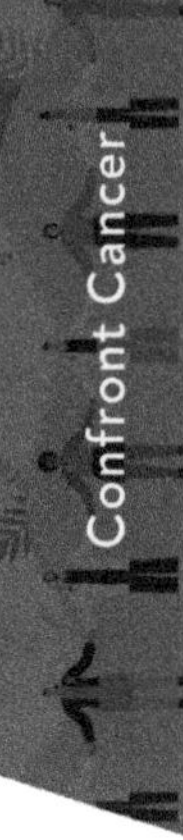

a single cell, the metastatic tumor may have a slightly different genetic makeup than the original.

Why does this tumor evolution matter in the context of metastasis and diagnosis? To diagnose cancer, the doctor must take a sample from one of the tumors. The tumor that is most easily accessible is the one that will be sampled (in order to minimize discomfort and complications), so they may biopsy one of the metastatic sites rather than the original tumor. These metastatic cells still have broadly similar genetic alterations and a microscopic appearance as the primary tumor. So, even if you have a biopsy from a metastatic tumor, the laboratory will likely detect that it came from the primary location, and this would be reflected in your diagnosis. For example, you may have a liver biopsy and be diagnosed with lung cancer. The critical point, though, is that if you have a biopsy from a metastatic site, some of the genetic alterations in that tumor might not be in the other tumors in your body, meaning that some treatments—primarily the targeted therapies—may work better on specific lesions and not others.

Let's look at this in the context of a patient who has lung cancer with a single genetic alteration in the protein EGFR, which we'll call mutation 1. The patient is treated first with an EGFR inhibitor, and due to the pressure that the treatment puts on the cancer cells, some of them develop a second EGFR mutation (mutation 2). These cells can grow even during treatment with the EGFR inhibitor, because their new mutation prevents the drug from acting on them.

The treatment will kill some cells in the primary tumor (those with mutation 1 only), but the cells with the new mutation will survive. Then let's say one cell with mutation 2 breaks off from the tumor and migrates to the liver to form a new tumor. All the cells of this metastatic tumor now have mutation 2 and therefore are resistant to the prescribed EGFR inhibitor. Thus, while the patient is taking the prescribed EGFR inhibitor, the liver tumor grows, while cells without mutation 2 are dying at the lung site, causing the lung tumor to shrink. Once this is detected, the patient may have another biopsy, which shows mutation 2. The doctor then switches to a different EGFR inhibitor that will work against the cells with mutation 1 *and* mutation 2.

Cancer is complicated, right? It is sometimes a wonder it doesn't happen more often given the thirty trillion cells in our bodies, some growing and dividing, some exposed to toxic chemicals and environments. Be grateful for that. For now, though, let's focus on how this basic knowledge of cancer can help you get the best diagnosis.

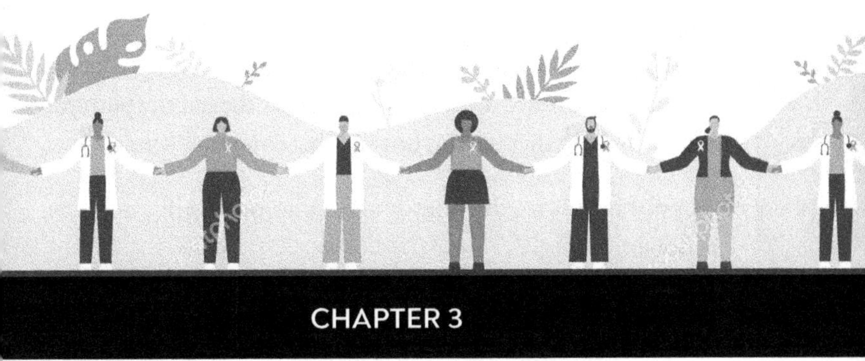

CHAPTER 3

DIAGNOSING CANCER

The doctor will begin by looking at the bigger picture of your cancer. Some of this will involve you sitting in a scanner as it takes images of your body. There will be poking and prodding. There will be questions about your lifestyle, and you and your family's medical history. There will be blood tests. Since you will spend time and undergo some discomfort for these procedures, it makes sense to find out why you're having them. The main procedures we'll look at in this chapter are imaging (taking pictures of your tumor) and biopsy (taking samples of your tumor).

TUMOR IMAGING

The doctor looks at body images to see where the primary cancer is and whether it has spread to other regions of the body. Later in the treatment process, they will take more images to see whether the treatment is working (i.e., to check if the tumor is getting smaller). The procedures that create images

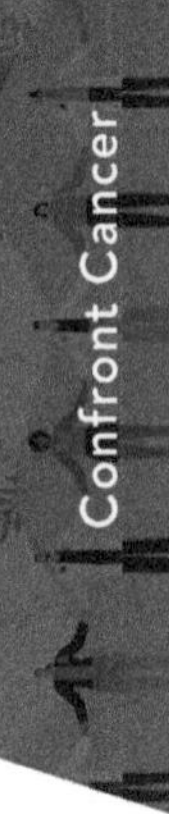

do this by sending energy, such as x-rays or magnetic fields, through your body. Your body then alters the energy pattern, which makes a picture you can see on a computer screen.

At your first scan, the doctor and radiologist will assess the following things:

- Does it look like cancer, or could something else be causing your symptoms?
- How large is the tumor—and therefore how long are you likely to have had it?
- Where does the tumor(s) lie in the body? Is the region complex or simple in terms of accessing it for tumor sampling or removal?
- Has the tumor spread to other parts of the body? Such spread usually suggests your cancer is stage IV, and you may need more aggressive treatment. Tumors in certain parts of the body may also indicate a more aggressive or hard-to-treat cancer.

Later on, your doctor and radiologist will take new images and will ask these questions:

- Has the tumor(s) shrunk in size compared with earlier images? In other words, is there evidence that the treatment is working?
- Are there any new tumors?

Following an effective cancer treatment, the doctor may perform further regular scans to check whether the tumor has returned.

At your diagnosis and periodically throughout your treatment, the doctor will image your tumors using various methods. The following is a description of each kind.

X-RAYS

You may have had an x-ray if you have broken a bone or when you've visited the dentist. An x-ray is a low-cost, fast scan that passes small amounts of electromagnetic radiation through your body. Electromagnetic radiation is similar to visible light but shorter in wavelength. x-rays can travel through most objects, including the body, and the rate at which they pass depends on the object's density. Bone structures are very dense, and this is why you get an x-ray when doctors suspect you may have broken a bone. A dye may provide a contrast for these scans and can be swallowed or injected before the procedure. These scans emit a small amount of **ionizing radiation**. Although small doses are considered safe, exposure to a lot of ionizing radiation can cause cancer, so it is sensible to keep the number of x-rays you have to a minimum, and they are usually avoided when possible in pregnant women. The amount of ionizing radiation from a single x-ray is not something you should worry about, though, and it is worth the exposure for the information the scan provides. Because x-rays are cheap and

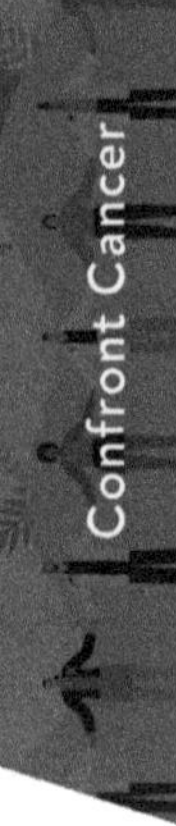

quick, you may have one before you have another type of scan to quickly provide information on your tumor(s).

CT SCAN

A computed tomography (CT) scan uses multiple x-rays to produce 3-D images of your body and tumor(s). The doctor applies 2-D x-rays from different angles, and then a 3-D image is generated by a computer. Certain CT scans require uptake of a dye before the scan. A "total body scan" will include at least your chest, stomach, and pelvis, and is usually used to see if other tumors are in your body. Other areas that may be scanned individually by CT are the head, neck, arms, and legs.

Because a CT scan uses x-rays that emit ionizing radiation, it is important to limit the number of CT scans and x-rays you have over time to reduce the risk of causing cancer.

MRI SCAN

A magnetic resonance imaging (MRI) scan uses strong radio waves to generate detailed images of your body and tumor. You may have seen the machines on TV—they are a long cylinder with a hole in the middle. You lie on a moving bed, which transports you into the cylinder for scanning. First, a magnet forces protons (a component of atoms) in the body to align with a magnetic field. A radiofrequency is then pulsed, and this excites the protons so they pull against the magnetic field. Once the radiofrequency stops, sensors can detect the release of energy and generate an image from it.

MRI scans are best on non-bony or soft tissue parts of the body. These scans do not emit ionizing radiation like a CT scan or x-ray does, so they are suitable for scanning reproductive organs and are safe for pregnant women.

ULTRASOUND

You may have encountered ultrasound during pregnancy. There's no exposure to ionizing radiation in ultrasound tests, meaning it's safe to use and is a great way to see a baby before it is born. Ultrasound scans use high-frequency sound waves to generate an image. These sound waves are not different from those we hear, except they are at a frequency that humans cannot detect. The waves are applied to your body and reflect to a transducer that transforms them into an image. The sound waves reflect off normal and cancerous tissue differently, helping doctors detect a possible tumor. Ultrasound is quicker to perform than many other types of scans and can image specific body regions that don't show up well by x-ray. Specifically, ultrasound is a very effective way of distinguishing solid tumors from fluid-filled cysts.

PET SCAN

A positron emission tomography (PET) scan uses a tracer agent that can be injected, swallowed, or inhaled. The tracer collects in organs or areas of the body that have higher chemical activity. Because cancer cells have a higher chemical activity than other cells, tumors will show up as bright spots on the PET scan.

TUMOR BIOPSY

Once you have had a scan of your tumor and your doctor knows where it is in your body, they may request a biopsy. A biopsy is a removal of some of the tumor cells that scientists can test in the laboratory to find out what type of cancer you have. If you have cancer of the blood (leukemia), the doctor will take a sample of your blood or bone marrow instead.

A tissue sample can be taken from almost any area of the body; the type of sample taken and the procedure to collect it will depend on where the tumor is and what type of cancer you may have. For example, a brain tumor biopsy is a lot more complicated than a skin tumor biopsy because of the differences in accessibility. The procedure may involve the acquisition of a tiny sample of cells (biopsy) or an attempted removal of the entire tumor (termed excisional biopsy or **resection**). Many oncologists can take a small sample, whereas a surgeon is needed to perform a resection.

NEEDLE BIOPSIES

A needle biopsy is a procedure in which a thin, hollow needle is inserted into your body and attached to a syringe that draws up a small piece of tissue or fluid from the tumor. The doctor guides the needle by feeling for the tumor or using a scan, if the tumor is deep inside the body. There are two types of needle biopsies:

- **Fine needle aspiration** uses a skinny needle of about 1.5 mm or less in diameter. A drug can be applied to the area before the procedure to make it numb (local anesthesia) prior to inserting the needle. The main advantage of fine needle aspiration is that the skin is not cut with a knife, and they can perform the procedure with minimal special preparation. Sometimes it's possible to make a diagnosis on the same day.

- **Core biopsy** involves removing a small cylinder of tissue of about 2 mm in diameter and at least a centimeter in length. It's a bit like coring an apple. The needles used in a core biopsy are slightly larger than those used in fine needle aspirates. A doctor in an outpatient clinic can perform a core biopsy. As with fine needle aspiration, a local anesthetic is used to numb the area, and an imaging scan can guide the biopsy or the doctor may be able to feel the tumor. The processing of a core biopsy can take longer than that of a fine needle aspirate, so you may not receive the results as quickly. However, it ensures that there will likely be enough tissue to perform the required tests.

EXCISIONAL OR INCISIONAL BIOPSIES

An excisional or incisional biopsy needs to be performed by a surgeon. The surgeon uses a local anesthetic and then cuts through the skin to remove the entire tumor (excisional biopsy) or a small part of the tumor (incisional biopsy). If the tumor is in a region that's difficult to access, such as inside the chest, stomach, or head, the patient is given a **general anesthetic** so they will feel no pain.

ENDOSCOPIC BIOPSY

Endoscopic biopsy is where a tissue sample is taken during an investigative test called an **endoscopy**. This involves the use of a tool called an endoscope, a thin, flexible, illuminated tube with a camera at the end. This tube is inserted into an organ or cavity, allowing the doctor to see the tumor. A cutting tool is also attached to the end of the endoscope so that tissue samples can be taken during the procedure. There are different types of endoscopes used to look at specific parts of the body. For example, a colonoscope is used to view the inside of the colon during a colonoscopy, and a bronchoscope is used to view the inside of the lung during a bronchoscopy.

SKIN BIOPSIES

There are several procedures that take a biopsy of the skin, and the one recommended for you depends on what type of skin tumor you likely have. If the tumor is on the outer layer of skin, a biopsy may be taken by shaving some of the tissue off; this procedure may be sufficient for a basal cell or squamous cell skin cancer. In other cases, it may take a **punch biopsy** or excisional biopsy to remove some of the deeper layers of the skin. This is required for melanoma, where it is important to know how deep into the skin the tumor has infiltrated.

LYMPH NODE BIOPSY

The **lymphatic system** is a network of tissues, vessels, and organs that move a colorless, watery liquid called **lymph** into the blood circulation. A lymph node looks like a kidney bean and is filled with white blood cells, the main cells of the immune system. There are hundreds of lymph nodes in the body, primarily in the neck, armpits, groin, belly, and chest. All materials and cells passing through a certain region of tissue have to pass through specific lymph nodes to filter out any harmful substances. When you have an infection, these lymph nodes fill up with cells and become hard or tender, which is why your mom may have checked for lumps in your neck when you were sick.

Tumor cells may hijack the lymphatic system, using it as a means of transport to other organs of the body. We see this especially in melanomas and breast cancers. The specific lymph node that is filtering the tumor site is likely the first place the tumor will go, so it is important to map which lymph node this is and remove it for biopsy. To find the specific lymph node(s) draining the tumor, the doctor will inject a small amount of a tracer material into the tumor region and then check lymph nodes to see whether the tracer is present. When a specific node is identified, it is removed, and the biopsy sample is sent to the laboratory. If that lymph node does not contain cancer cells, no more lymph nodes will need to be removed, because it's unlikely the cancer has spread. However, if they find cancer cells in this lymph node, other lymph nodes in the area will also be removed and examined.

WHAT HAPPENS AFTER THE BIOPSY?

Once you have had a biopsy, the sample is taken to the laboratory where tests are performed on it. The pathology laboratory specializes in examination of human tissues to diagnose disease and will conduct the first tests. The pathology testing on your biopsy will most likely occur either at a laboratory at the hospital where you had the sample taken or at another hospital close by. The scientists and doctors at the pathology laboratory (pathologists) are highly trained and can easily define which cancer you have based on the cell pattern, shape, and staining.

Preparation of the tumor for pathology and genetic diagnosis usually involves fixing the tissue using a preservative. This fixation preserves the genetic material and structure of the tissue. Fixing occurs by immersing the tissue in a weak form of formaldehyde and then dehydrating it. They then embed the dehydrated tissue in a block of wax that completely covers the tissue. In this form, the tissue is stable for many years and can be returned to for further testing. For analysis, the wax block is shaved into thin slices called *sections*, which are then mounted onto glass slides to allow visualization under the microscope. Some of the tissue that is removed in the biopsy may not be tumor tissue; it could be the surrounding normal tissue, or it could be immune cells and blood vessels. In most cases, the report you get back from the laboratory will tell you the percentage of the specimen that was tumor.

Because thin sections of natural tissues don't show up very well under the microscope, scientists usually stain them with chemicals before examining them. The pathology laboratory will examine almost all tumors using a stain typically referred to as an H&E stain, which is a combination of two stains: hematoxylin and eosin. Hematoxylin stains the part of the cell containing the genetic material (the nucleus) blue, and eosin stains the jelly-like liquid that makes up the rest of the cell (the cytoplasm) pink, with other structures around the cells taking on different shades and combinations of these colors. The stain shows the general pattern of the cells and gives an overview of tissue and cell structure that provides information such as how fast the cells may be dividing, where they may have come from, and their function.

Let's look at this using an example from a lung tumor specimen. The pathologist will look under the microscope at the cells stained with H&E and may see cells containing a large amount of pink cytoplasm that are different sizes or shapes. The blue nucleus may be very dark, and there could be some connections between the cells. We see this pattern in squamous cell carcinoma of the lung, and that would likely be the pathologist's diagnosis. Alternatively, they may see cells with a large amount of cytoplasm but also a large nucleus containing granules or cysts. This pattern is likely a lung adenocarcinoma. Alternatively, and more rarely, some pockets of cells may look like squamous cell carcinoma, while other areas look like adenocarcinoma, or the cells may not look much like either type, which makes the diagnosis difficult to define.

Depending on what type of tumor you have, the cells may be stained to identify specific proteins using a process called **immunohistochemistry** (IHC). This method uses antibodies linked to a fluorescent marker to tag proteins in a tissue sample. After the antibodies bind to the protein, the fluorescence is activated, and the location of the protein in the tissue can then be observed under a microscope. IHC is used to inform the diagnosis of most cancers. One very common example is the detection of the HER2 protein in breast cancer. An antibody specific to HER2 is used to identify tumors that have high expression levels of this protein. Patients with HER2-positive tumors will greatly benefit from treatment with a HER2 inhibitor such as Herceptin.

The other type of testing the doctors should perform on your biopsy is a genetic test, which may identify genetic alterations present in your tumor that will refine your diagnosis. There's more detail about genetic testing in Chapter 4.

When the necessary tests have been done, the remainder of the tumor biopsy will be stored. The amount remaining will depend on the original yield from the biopsy, the number of tests that have been performed, and the amount of tissue required for the tests. For example, if you had a fine needle aspirate, which yields just a small number of cells, there is likely to be little, if any, material remaining after the tests. If some of the tissue is stored, your doctor may return to it at later stages in your disease to find more options for treatment. It is also possible for the remaining material to be stored for future scientific research, for which you would be asked to provide consent.

If some of the tissue is stored, your doctor may return to it at later stages in your disease to find more options for treatment.

Once your pathology and genetic reports are available, your doctor will collate the information to make a final diagnosis. If the case is complex or difficult to diagnose, the doctor could take the details to a multidisciplinary team of pathologists, geneticists, oncologists, and surgeons, who will discuss all aspects of your tumor and determine the diagnosis and what the optimal treatment should be. It is important to note, however, that these decisions can only be made based on the tests that have been performed.

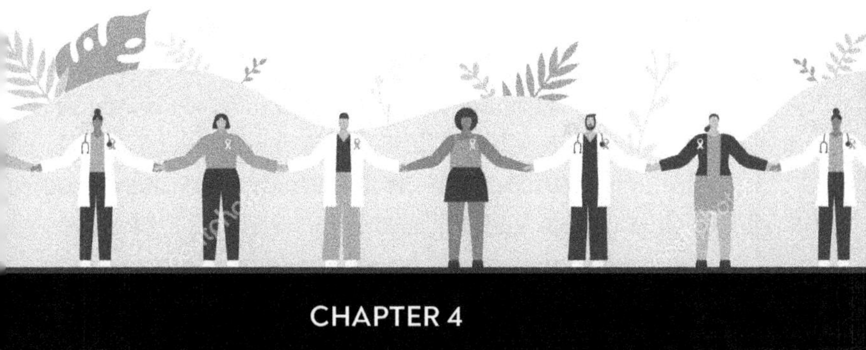

CHAPTER 4

GENETIC TESTS AND SAMPLES

The other type of testing that the doctors should perform on your biopsy sample is a genetic test, which will refine your diagnosis and possibly identify genetic alterations present in your tumor. In this chapter, we will look at these genetic tests and how you can find out more about the mutations in your tumor.

Historically, the diagnosis of your tumor and the treatment options you received would have been based on how your cells looked under the microscope (pathology). Increasingly, though, as we learn more about the genetics of certain tumors and which genetic alterations respond to which drugs, the diagnosis of cancer is based on the genetic alterations present in a particular tumor.

Even more recently, regulatory bodies have approved drugs based solely on a genetic alteration in a tumor and not at all determined by the tumor's pathology or site of origin. For example, if your tumor has been found to have a rearrangement of a gene called NTRK, you will be given an NTRK inhibitor, regardless of where in the body your cancer arose or what its cells look like under the microscope. However, you would only know that you have one of these genetic alterations if you have a test for that gene. As NTRK rearrangements are rare, they are usually only detected by the use of a broad genetic test.

Broad genetic tests include comprehensive sequencing of up to three hundred genes. Compared with single-gene tests, they are costly, use more of your specimen, and can take longer for the result (about two weeks versus three to seven days for testing of a single gene). These types of tests can be applied to many different cancer types and provide a lot more information on your tumor. They are usually performed at a centralized location, either a very large university hospital or a private provider, such as Foundation Medicine and Caris Life Sciences. Your local lab will prepare the specimen in a wax block, and then fine slivers of the block will be shaved off and mounted onto glass microscope slides. These slides, along with an H&E-stained slide, will be sent to the private provider's pathologist, who will assess which parts of the specimen are the tumor using the stained slide and then shave off the corresponding portion of the other slides into a tube; this material will be used to perform the test. After running the test, the pathologist will provide a report to your doctor that includes details of the genetic alterations in your tumor and the recommended treatment options.

Large private centers most often perform the broad genetic tests, while community hospitals tend to provide smaller tests performed by the hospital laboratory itself or at a nearby hospital.

GENETIC TESTS FOR TUMORS

The basis of all genetic testing done on tumors is that some of the tumor cells' genetic material (**DNA** or **RNA**) is extracted and analyzed. Traditionally, this is done by taking a tumor biopsy (as we discussed in Chapter 3) and growing the cells in the laboratory, then analyzing the chromosomes or genes from the cultured cells. This is an invasive method of testing, and obtaining a sample from the tumor carries some risk. It also requires an appointment with a special doctor who is qualified to take the biopsy. Despite this, it is still the most common method for finding information on your tumor.

CIRCULATING TUMOR DNA

Over the past decade, there has been a push for diagnostic tests that don't involve such invasive procedures in order to spare patients the discomfort and risk of having to have a biopsy needle or knife inserted into their body. One of these tests, sometimes referred to as **liquid biopsy**, detects tumor DNA in your blood to determine whether you have cancer and what genetic alterations your cancer has. A number of blood tests have been approved for this purpose, and all of them fall into the broad sequencing panel group, with twenty to five hundred genes sequenced to provide a comprehensive genetic profile of your tumor. A blood sample is a much more comfortable procedure than a biopsy and can be taken in a community clinic, whereas a biopsy often requires your attendance at a more specialized clinic.

If your doctor orders one of these blood tests, you will need to have your blood drawn. The blood sample will be spun very quickly in a machine called a centrifuge. Essentially, this process can be likened to separating the curds from whey in milk. When milk is spun at a high force, the liquid (whey) separates from the solid proteins (curds). A similar effect happens with your blood. With a sufficiently forceful spin, the cells in your blood will separate from the liquid (plasma). The plasma, which contains pieces of DNA, can then be sent to the sequencing center for tests.

Why does your plasma contain pieces of DNA? Well, DNA can be shed from healthy cells and enter your blood circulation. Inflamed tissue may shed more DNA, because some of its cells are being destroyed and pieces of DNA will be released from that process. Tumor cells shed DNA by both processes, and the amount released can increase as the disease advances. The amount of circulating tumor DNA (ctDNA) shed into the blood can also depend on the location of your tumor. For example, a tumor in the brain releases less DNA into the blood because the brain has a tight protective mechanism preventing the movement of substances into and out of its tissues.

I have mentioned some advantages of the ctDNA test based on logistics around taking the sample, but they also offer another important advantage, which is related to the results you get back. As DNA is shed from all tumors in the body, genetic blood tests can detect genetic alterations from any tumor that is present. This is important because, as we mentioned in Chapter 2, some tumor cells may have additional genetic alterations from those collected by a traditional tumor biopsy, and these cells could be resistant to certain therapies. A solid biopsy takes a small piece of tissue from one tumor in your body (usually the most accessible one), and the genetic test provides a comprehensive genetic profile, *but only of that biopsied tissue*. You would not get information about the other parts of that tumor or any other tumors, and some of these other malignant areas may have genetic alterations that indicate you should not have a specific therapy. Testing the blood may provide this information, because it is potentially testing pieces of DNA shed from any tumor in your body.

There are limitations to blood tests, though, and because of this, I always advocate for both a ctDNA test and a tumor biopsy test to gain the most information. In some cases, the amount of ctDNA shed from the tumor is too little to determine the full genetic profile of your tumor. This is more likely when you are in the early stages of disease or if you have a very small tumor. If you have one of these tests and the level of shedding is low, you will likely need to have a biopsy, anyway.

Two of the most prominent centers that test ctDNA are Guardant Health and Foundation Medicine. The results of these tests usually take a few weeks to come back. The decision to use one of these tests must balance how much information you can get out of it with when the results will come in. Ask your doctor these questions:

- Are there likely to be mutations detected that will guide my treatment options?
- Will the results come back quickly enough that I can start treatment when needed?

GERMLINE GENETIC TESTING

Germline genetics have nothing to do with germs! Germ cells are your sex cells: sperm in males and eggs in females. So, **germline** genetics relates to the genetic material that is passed from generation to generation. This material is present in every cell of our bodies and provides a blueprint for our physical form and behavior. The variations in our germline create the family characteristics that were passed from our grandparents to our parents to us.

Germline mutations are also passed from generation to generation. Because these mutations sometimes affect genes that are associated with the development of cancer, some families have more individuals with specific cancers than would be expected. An example of this is a genetic alteration of a gene called BRCA1 (BReast CAncer gene). We all have the BRCA1 gene, which plays a very important role in helping to repair DNA damage that can cause and develop cancers. But in some people, the BRCA gene does not work properly due to a genetic mutation. This affects the ability of their cells to repair DNA that has been damaged, causing more acquired genetic alterations to build up, which can initiate and accelerate the development of breast cancer. An alteration such as this can be passed down through generations, elevating the risk of breast cancer in individuals who inherit it.

When the genetic profile of a tumor sample is analyzed, both the germline alterations and the acquired alterations will be detected. In most cases, the genetic alterations used for a cancer diagnosis are acquired. However, sometimes germline genetics may be important because some variations may increase your susceptibility to developing cancer.

It is possible to detect these familial genetic alterations in your tumor specimen because each cell is a part of you, and its underlying genetic makeup is the same as all the other (healthy) cells in your body. However, in a cancer specimen, it is sometimes difficult to distinguish whether an alteration arrived in your body in the germline—in other words, when you were conceived—or if it has been acquired during your lifetime.

Suppose doctors identify an important alteration in your tumor sample that is thought to be a germline mutation. In that case, you will need a confirmatory test to ensure that the alteration also exists in healthy cells; this test can usually be performed with a blood sample. If the confirmatory test on the blood sample is positive, you will be referred for genetic counseling. This will help you fully understand what this genetic alteration means for you and your family, and will allow you to determine whether you would like to disclose this information to members of your family.

Germline genetics is unrelated to the genetic alterations that we acquire throughout life—sometimes called **somatic mutations**—some of which may cause cancer. This acquisition of genetic alterations occurs at a steady rate as we age and can increase due to certain environmental exposures. For example, there may be an accelerated accumulation of genetic alterations in skin that is exposed to ultraviolet light or in lungs exposed to smoke. These acquired genetic alterations are not passed on to our offspring because they are not present within our germ cells.

CONSIDERATIONS FOR GENETIC TESTING

In deciding which tests should be performed on your biopsy or blood sample, the key factors your doctor will consider are

- how well the test identifies samples that are positive for the important features (the **sensitivity** of the test);
- how well the test identifies samples that are negative for the important features (the **specificity** of the test);
- whether there is enough tissue specimen for diagnosis and molecular testing;
- the invasiveness and risk of procedure (e.g., a blood sample is much less invasive than a lung biopsy);
- how easy it is to interpret the findings from the test;
- whether the results of the test will be available in time for you to start your treatment; and
- what technology and expertise are available (community hospitals usually have less technology and fewer resources than academic centers).

The type of test your doctor orders will depend on two factors: what kind of cancer you have and how quickly you need to get started on treatment (and therefore how quickly you need the test results back). Single-gene tests can be useful, as they are often performed on-site, they are less expensive, and they provide faster results. However, if the results come back negative, you will be left with limited options, and there may not be enough biopsy tissue left to perform further tests. Since some cancers have a very defined treatment protocol that is based on specific mutations only, running a test for up to five hundred genes is not cost effective, it will use up more of your specimen, and it will take longer than necessary. If your cancer has been termed *advanced* or *aggressive*, it is important that you start treatment as quickly as possible, so a test that will provide rapid results is likely the most appropriate in that situation.

Another factor is your doctor's accessibility to these tests. Many big academic hospitals have their own large sequencing laboratories, reducing the cost and the time it takes to receive results. A doctor in a small community hospital, however, will not have access to these genetic sequencing tests, and in order to perform a large sequencing panel, your biopsy will need to be sent to one of the large sequencing vendors, which can add cost. This lack of testing is a real problem. A 2019 survey showed that only 22 percent of patients with lung cancer were tested for the four recommended genetic alterations outside of academic hospitals. Sixty-five percent of health care professionals

Sixty-five percent of health care professionals reported that a patient's insurance coverage factored into their decision to order diagnostic tests.

reported that a patient's insurance coverage factored into their decision to order diagnostic tests, and 45 percent said that the patient's out-of-pocket expenses could mean that they don't prescribe the targeted therapy.

A final factor to consider is the amount of tumor that was removed for testing. If a small biopsy was taken (e.g., a fine needle aspirate), there are limited tests that can be performed on that tissue, and maximizing the success of genetic tests on that material is essential. Therefore, using a test that requires smaller pieces of tissue will be optimal.

Hopefully, this chapter and the previous one have convinced you that the investigational procedures for your diagnosis will not be as harrowing as you previously thought. All of them have a purpose, and some are better suited to you and your situation than others. Once you have had the tests done, you then need to interpret the results.

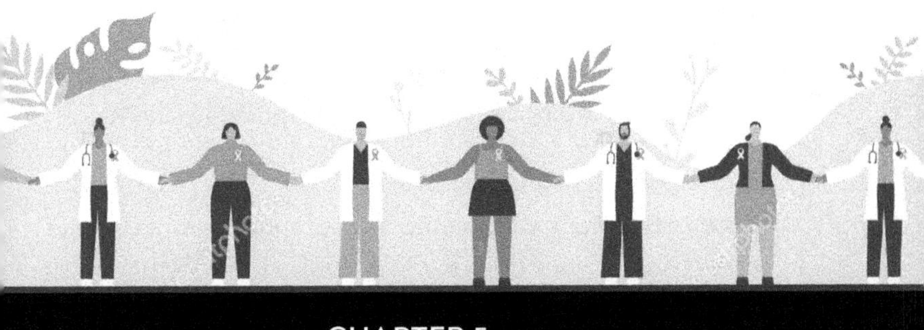

CHAPTER 5

UNDERSTANDING YOUR TEST RESULTS

Once the genetic and pathology tests on your tumor specimen are complete and you have had all your scans, your doctor will make a final diagnosis. If the diagnosis is complicated, the health care team will discuss these reports at a multidisciplinary team meeting. Then you will be given a definitive diagnosis at your appointment with your doctor.

Now the hard part: you have all the results of your tests back, and your doctor has provided you with a diagnosis. Most people would take that diagnosis and leave it to the doctor to propose options for treatment. Don't do this. I'm not saying you should distrust your doctor, but cancer is complicated, and new medical and diagnostic advances are coming out all the time. It is impossible for the doctor to know everything about every cancer. In 2020, they updated the United States' clinical cancer guidelines eight times! It's no wonder that in a survey of health professionals, one in four doctors did not know about the updated policies.

It is essential to discuss how your doctor arrived at this diagnosis to fully understand any complications with your case. Usually, your doctor will provide this information to you without you having to ask for it, but there may be some information that you have to ask for specifically. Once you have had this discussion, you can also ask your doctor for the genetic, pathology, and radiology reports they used to arrive at the diagnosis, which are helpful to keep as a record. Read those reports and try to understand as much as you can. Bring the information to your consultations, so that you will be in the best position to discuss what you have found.

The reason you need to discuss your diagnosis with the doctor is to get an idea of how confident they are in their diagnosis. All your treatment options will hinge on this. If your diagnosis is clear-cut and your health care team is experienced with the type of cancer you have, you can be satisfied that the treatment options presented to you are the optimal ones available. These therapies have been thoroughly tested in clinical trials on tumors with features similar to yours.

For example, suppose you have lung cancer that clearly shows a lung adenocarcinoma pattern under the microscope, and the genetic test has identified an EGFR mutation. In that case, you can be confident of your diagnosis of EGFR-mutated lung adenocarcinoma, and your doctor can follow the specific pathway provided in the clinical guidelines for this subtype of tumor. However, if there is a discrepancy between the different laboratory findings and the wrong diagnosis is made, the treatment options presented to you may not be very effective. An example is if parts of your lung tumor look like squamous cell carcinoma under the microscope, while other parts look like adenocarcinoma. The laboratory scientists and doctors will do their best to categorize your tumor, but it is important to understand that a diagnosis of lung adenocarcinoma under these circumstances is not as precise as in the first example.

Another part of the discussion with your doctor should include which tests were performed and how much of your tumor is left for further testing. Your diagnosis is based solely on the results that come back from your tests and scans. You can discuss and understand the rationale behind why your doctor ordered those specific tests and, if the diagnosis is not a clear one, whether you have options for further testing to confirm the diagnosis. Even if it is not beneficial to have more comprehensive testing at this time, it could be helpful in the future if you need to stop the first treatment and start another.

Once you and your doctor have thoroughly discussed why you had specific tests, you can obtain the reports that came back from each laboratory and assess them for yourself. This chapter is primarily to guide you in understanding what these reports mean and how the information can have a bearing on your treatment.

There are several sites, both within hospitals and private, where testing can be performed. The reports from each of these laboratories look slightly different. In all cases, the report will include the names of the gene(s) that were tested (usually capitalized: e.g., EGFR, NTRK). If a mutation in a gene was found, that will be stated in the main body of the report.

LABORATORY REPORTS

Every time one of your samples is sent to a laboratory for testing, the laboratory sends your doctor a report stating the results of the test. If your doctor or patient portal does not provide you with that report, ask for it, as it will provide you with complete information. These are the sections to check on every report:

If your doctor or patient portal does not provide you with that report, ask for it, as it will provide you with complete information.

Name and date of birth: check to make sure this test result is yours!

Date of sample collection: This is important because, throughout the course of your different treatments, you may have many biopsies. This will let you know which biopsy they tested.

Tests performed: This is important so you know what genes have been tested. For example, you may have had a test of a single gene, such as EGFR, in which case you will not know about mutations in other genes. It also allows you to look up that test and see whether it is reputable (it usually will be) and what the sensitivity and specificity of the test are.

The result of your test: this could be positive protein markers on immunohistochemistry, mutations found on a genomic report, or features seen on a pathology report.

Interpretation of the results: Most test reports will offer some sort of interpretation to suggest what the results mean. This information must be considered along with all the other test results you have on your tumor at that point in time. Some reports will even suggest which drugs may be appropriate.

You can find an example genomic test report on Foundation Medicine's website in the Useful Links section.

FAILED TESTS

It is possible that one test on your specimen will fail or produce an inconclusive result. This failure could be due to issues with sampling, storage, transit, or analysis of the specimen. For a successful test, the doctor must collect an appropriate amount of sample in the correct tube containing the appropriate transport solution, and they must ensure it is promptly transported to the laboratory. In some cases, errors or unfortunate circumstances compromise the sample at one of these steps. There can also be issues with the analysis of the sample at the receiving laboratory. These issues can be technical, such as a compromised machine or reagent, or truly biological. One instance of this is the presence of a specific genetic alteration in just a few cells of the tumor, meaning that the test produces results that cannot be confirmed as positive or negative. In each of these cases, they will issue a report indicating that the test produced an inconclusive result. If you have a sufficient amount of biopsy tissue stored, it may be possible to rerun these tests, assuming the material was stored appropriately.

GETTING A SECOND OPINION

The following are questions you can ask your doctor to stimulate discussion around your diagnosis:

- How was this diagnosis determined?
- How sure are you that my diagnosis is accurate?
- Do all the tests—scans, pathology, and genetics—point to the same diagnosis?
- If there is doubt, are there further tests I can have to confirm the diagnosis?

Seeking a second opinion may delay your treatment, and this is an important factor to consider. In almost all situations, though, it is well worth a reasonable delay in treatment to ensure your diagnosis has been properly evaluated, especially if your doctor does not have much experience with the type of cancer you have. You should speak to your doctor about this, as they will have to send your medical records to any other doctor who sees you.

Do not worry you will upset your doctor by seeking a second opinion. I was helping a friend figure out the diagnosis of her relative's pancreatic cancer a while ago, and I suggested they have a ctDNA test done to help identify new options for treatment when all the obvious options had been exhausted. When they asked the doctor for the test, the doctor took a saliva sample and sent it to a company called Invitae for a genetic test. Unfortunately, this test, although linked to cancer, is a germline test like the ones we mentioned in Chapter 4; it identifies whether your germline genetics increase your likelihood of getting cancer, rather than diagnosing cancer. This was a completely inappropriate test, but because the doctor was not familiar with ctDNA testing, it was ordered and came back negative. This kind of error is misleading for the patient and can be avoided with a second opinion.

Do not worry you will upset your doctor by seeking a second opinion.

Cancer is a complex and serious disease, and it is best managed by teams of experts who are up-to-date with the latest advances. New advancements in cancer therapy are happening so quickly that it's practically impossible for every doctor to be up-to-date on every aspect of every subtype of the disease.

The best place to seek a second opinion is at a hospital designated as a Cancer Center or Comprehensive Cancer Center by the National Cancer Institute (see the Useful Links section). At these hospitals, the doctors have high levels of expertise and specialize in particular types of cancers. You want to find a doctor at one of these centers who has many years of experience treating your specific type of cancer. Search your health insurance website to find a list of doctors. To find out if a doctor is appropriately qualified, you can look up where they trained and what they are certified for (see the Useful Links section). In addition, the doctor may be a member of specific cancer societies, such as the American Society of Clinical Oncology. Find out how many years of experience the doctor has treating your type of cancer. There's more information about getting a second opinion in Chapter 8.

Analyzing the reports from the tests on your tumor can be complicated, but you have the information and resources in this book to help. The point is to work with your health care team to find the right diagnosis. Don't just trust—question. Take a seat at the table; you are the person these decisions will affect the most.

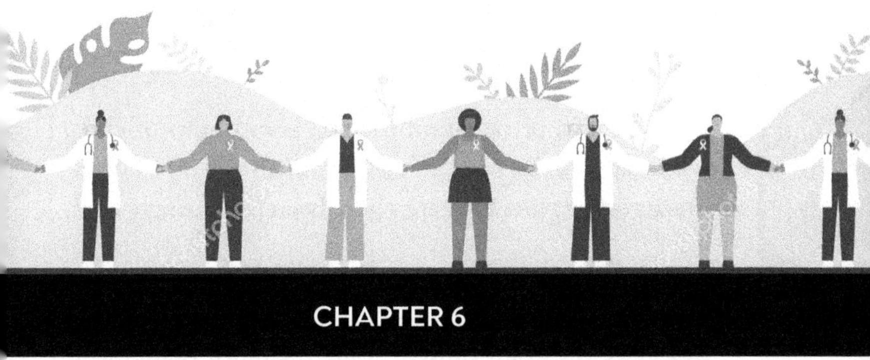

CHAPTER 6

CANCER THERAPY

TYPES OF THERAPY

Depending on the type and stage of cancer you have, your doctors will likely offer you one or more kinds of therapy. These may include traditional approaches, newer targeted treatments, or a combination of both. Let's have a more detailed look at these therapies and the circumstances where they might be used.

TRADITIONAL THERAPIES

CHEMOTHERAPY

Chemotherapy is any treatment where powerful chemicals are given to you by mouth or intravenously (directly into your bloodstream) to kill rapidly growing cells in your body, such as cancer cells. Chemotherapy includes targeted therapy, which is further discussed below.

RADIOTHERAPY

Radiotherapy, or radiation therapy, uses beams of energy to kill cancer cells. Most often, this involves x-rays, but protons or other types of energy have been increasingly used.

In most cases, the high-energy beams come from an external machine that aims the beams at the tumor, but in some cases, they place the beam emitter inside the body. Radiotherapy kills cancer cells by damaging their genetic material. It can also kill healthy cells, but by carefully targeting the beam at the tumor, side effects to healthy cells can be minimized. In addition, healthy cells can often repair this type of damage.

SURGERY

Surgery is the oldest type of cancer treatment, in which a surgeon removes the tumor and nearby tissue. It is highly effective for many types of cancer, and in some cases can completely remove the tumor with no further need for treatment. In other cases, the tumor may be too tightly intertwined with important healthy cells to be removed.

TARGETED THERAPIES

As we have seen, we can further define cancers using genetic tests, and that is informative for treatment. That's because determining the pathological and genetic features of an individual's cancer allows the personalization of their treatment: so-called **personalized medicine**. To illustrate, let's return to a specific type of lung cancer we've already mentioned: EGFR-mutant lung cancer.

Around 15 percent of lung cancers have an alteration in a protein called EGFR. The alteration (mutation) arises in the gene that provides the cells with instructions to make this protein. This mutated protein allows the cancer cells to grow uncontrollably, rather than in the tightly controlled fashion in which most cell growth is regulated. EGFR alterations are more often seen in non-smokers and younger patients, and in Asia. This suggests that the factors that increase your risk for EGFR-mutant cancer differ from those of other lung cancers, which tend to arise through heavy smoking.

The discovery of EGFR mutations in lung cancer led to many drugs designed to target that protein, called EGFR inhibitors. As you might expect, clinical trials showed that patients with an EGFR mutation in their lung cancer responded better to EGFR inhibitors. For this reason, lung cancer patients need to know whether their tumor has an EGFR mutation.

Drugs that directly inhibit an aberrant cancer protein brought significant improvements to traditional chemotherapeutic agents. The reason for this is that chemotherapy targets all rapidly dividing cells of the body (including normal cells), and this causes side effects such as vomiting, nausea, fatigue, and hair loss. Targeted agents like EGFR inhibitors preferentially target the tumor cells because only these cells have altered EGFR; normal cells don't. The result is fewer side effects and more effective targeting.

chemotherapy targets all rapidly dividing cells of the body (including normal cells), and this causes side effects such as vomiting, nausea, fatigue, and hair loss.

Let's dig deeper into how targeted therapies for cancer differ from conventional chemotherapy. Conventional chemotherapy is the most well-known type of treatment for cancer. It leads to the loss of hair and the pale appearance that is often depicted in the movies in patients with cancer—for example, *My Sister's Keeper*, which was adapted from the best-selling book by Jodi Picoult. In that movie, a young girl has leukemia and is treated with conventional chemotherapy. Her mother shaves off her own hair in solidarity with her daughter, who is losing her hair due to the treatment. The reason conventional chemotherapy causes hair loss is that it kills not only tumor cells, but any cells that are rapidly growing—for example, those in your hair roots. Targeted therapies most often block tumor cell growth rather than kill the cells, and they are much more selective about the cells they act on. For this reason, they can give targeted therapy in much higher doses because it is less likely to induce significant side effects. Higher doses most often mean a more effective therapy. For all these reasons, targeted therapy is considered an important focus for drugs in development.

Several targeted therapies are approved by regulatory bodies worldwide, including the Medicines and Healthcare Products Regulatory Agency (MHRA) in the United Kingdom and the Food and Drug Administration (FDA) in the United States. More targeted therapies are in clinical trials right now.

There are six main types of targeted therapy. Let's deep dive into each one of them here.

MONOCLONAL ANTIBODIES

Monoclonal antibodies can deliver toxic molecules to the cancer cells, killing those cells specifically. An antibody is a protein that matches another protein. For cancer therapy, an antibody is attached to a toxic molecule, such as a radioactive substance or poisonous chemical, that kills the cell. By perfectly matching an antibody to a protein that is present on the cancer cells but not the normal cells, we can deliver the toxic molecules directly and specifically to the cancer cells. The antibody binds to the cancer cell, the toxic molecule linked to the antibody is taken up by the cancer cell, and the cell dies. The toxin will not affect normal cells because they lack the target for the antibody, and this minimizes side effects from the drug. The first monoclonal targeted antibody, trastuzumab, came out in 1998. Trastuzumab, also known as Herceptin, targets a protein called HER2, which is produced at high levels in some types of breast cancer. This type of breast cancer relies on HER2 for sustained growth; therefore, blocking the protein stunts the tumor's growth. Trastuzumab remains an essential component of treatment for breast cancers that are reliant on HER2 for their growth. It is now usually given alongside conventional chemotherapy but can also be given alone.

ANGIOGENESIS INHIBITORS

Angiogenesis inhibitors block the formation of new blood vessels, which occurs in certain diseases or during wound repair. Tumor cells require a connected blood supply to deliver oxygen and nutrients to support their growth. By destroying the blood vessels and blocking the blood supply to the tumor, angiogenesis inhibitors indirectly block tumor growth. The most commonly targeted angiogenesis signaling protein is vascular endothelial growth factor (VEGF). Bevacizumab was the first drug to target VEGF and is approved by the FDA for metastatic colorectal or renal cancer, glioblastoma, non-squamous non-small-cell lung cancer, and liver, epithelial ovarian, fallopian tube, and primary peritoneal cancers. Other angiogenesis inhibitors are available that target different molecules involved in angiogenesis.

APOPTOSIS INDUCERS

Apoptosis inducers stimulate a process by which cells undergo a controlled death, called **apoptosis**. Apoptosis is the way our bodies get rid of damaged or old cells. Cancer cells often harbor a lot of DNA damage and would usually be direct targets for apoptosis—but they hijack this process so they can avoid death. Apoptosis inducers aim to stimulate apoptosis and destroy the cancer cells. One recently approved apoptosis inducer is venetoclax, which doctors combine with conventional chemotherapy to treat acute myeloid leukemia. Venetoclax targets an anti-apoptosis protein called BCL2, preventing it from allowing cells to escape apoptosis.

HORMONE THERAPIES

Hormone therapies slow or stop the growth of cancers that require certain hormones in order to grow. Cancer can become addicted to one or more hormones that allow its cells to grow uncontrollably. Hormone therapies can hinder cancer growth by either stopping the body from producing the hormones or interfering with their action. The very first targeted cancer drug, tamoxifen, came out in the 1970s and was a type of hormone therapy. Tamoxifen prevents the action of estrogen, to which some breast cancers are highly addicted. The tamoxifen molecule is similar in size and shape to estrogen, and it binds to the estrogen docking site (the estrogen receptor, or ER) on breast cancer cells, excluding estrogen. By interfering with the ability of estrogen to stimulate breast cancer cell growth, tamoxifen provides an effective treatment option for patients with breast cancers that highly express the estrogen receptor. Now, multiple ER-targeting drugs are available, including anastrozole, exemestane, fulvestrant, letrozole, and toremifene.

IMMUNOTHERAPIES

Immunotherapies kick-start the immune system to recognize, target, and kill cancer cells. Our bodies have several layers of protection in place to prevent cancer from forming. This is essential given the enormous number of cells in the body, many of which are dividing. The first prominent protection mechanism identifies errors in the DNA and repairs them before the cell divides. If that fails, the second protection mechanism recognizes damaged cells and initiates apoptosis, as we discussed above.

Your immune system can also provide a third protection mechanism. In the same way that your immune cells recognize an infection and kill off the offending bacteria or virus, they can also recognize cells that have started to become different. When this happens, they kill those cells to prevent them from dividing and becoming cancerous. But cancer cells have developed mechanisms to "hide" from the immune system. Immunotherapies target these mechanisms—specific proteins that allow cancer cells to evade the immune system—which then kick-starts the immune system back into action and allows your own body to target and destroy the cancer cells. Pretty clever!

One type of immunotherapy inhibits a mechanism that cancer cells use to hide from the immune system, which involves a protein on their surface called programmed death ligand 1 (PD-L1). PD-L1 binds to killer cells of the immune system to tell them "Don't kill me." The killer cells detect this protein and leave the cancer cells alone, allowing them to grow uncontrollably. Drugs have been developed that bind to the PD-L1 docking site on the killer immune cells, called PD-1 (programmed cell death 1), and this prevents the killer cells from being affected by the high levels of PD-L1 on the cancer cells' surface. This means the killer cells then recognize the cancer cells as deviant and kill them. Pembrolizumab (Keytruda) and nivolumab (Opdivo) are common monoclonal antibodies that target this mechanism and are approved for many types of cancer.

There are several success stories with immunotherapy. I remember a friend going through multiple treatments for her cancer, none of which worked. Then she was put on a clinical trial for an immunotherapy drug. This drug cured her! It seemed like a miracle at the time, but this is only one of a huge number of success stories with these drugs.

SIGNAL TRANSDUCTION INHIBITORS

Signal transduction inhibitors (sometimes called tyrosine kinase inhibitors) hamper the way in which a cancer cell responds to signals from its environment. For example, some cancer cells can grow uncontrollably despite the presence of external "stop growing" signs. Signal transduction inhibitors work to shut down this inappropriate response by either targeting the protein on the cancer cell's surface that detects the signal or targeting a protein within the cell that is part of the **signaling cascade**. An example of a signal transduction inhibitor targeting a molecule within the cell is imatinib (Gleevec), which targets a genetic alteration that causes two proteins, BCR and ABL1, to become fused, making a new hybrid protein that causes chronic myeloid leukemia (CML). The BCR-ABL fusion was discovered over fifty years ago and was the first genetic alteration found to cause cancer. For this reason, imatinib is considered a landmark targeted drug. Every leukemic cell in a patient with CML has this fusion, and therefore, imatinib is highly effective for this cancer. Patients can remain on this drug effectively for many years.

WHAT ARE THE LIMITATIONS OF TARGETED THERAPIES?

Targeted therapies represent a great stride in the right direction for cancer treatment, but they have their own set of limitations. Because tremendous pressure is applied to cancer cells when a targeted therapy is given, many cancers evolve resistance mechanisms.

Resistance to targeted therapy was first described in lung cancer. Patients with lung tumors treated with the first EGFR inhibitor, gefitinib (Iressa), eventually stopped responding. It was discovered that this was due to their tumors developing an additional mutation in EGFR; this new genetic alteration prevented gefitinib from working. This discovery led to the development of second-generation inhibitors such as afatinib (Gilotrif) and dacomitinib (Vizimpro). Subsequent resistance to the second-generation inhibitors resulted in the development of third-generation inhibitors such as osimertinib (Tagrisso), the EGFR inhibitor that is most commonly prescribed today. One approach to avoid resistance is to administer targeted therapies in combination; for example, the targeted therapy trastuzumab is often used along with conventional chemotherapy to treat patients with breast cancer.

Another limitation of targeted therapy is the fact that some targets are challenging for drug development. One example of this is RAS, which was referred to as an "undruggable target" until relatively recently. There were no drugs available to target this protein, which acts within the cell after receiving specific cues from proteins on the surface, such as EGFR. With improved chemistry, however, drugs that can target this protein have begun to emerge.

Although targeted therapies aim to act on cancer cells specifically and they generally have fewer side effects than conventional chemotherapeutics, side effects such as blood clotting and wound healing problems, liver problems, high blood pressure, diarrhea, and rashes can still occur with these agents. Some of these side effects indicate response to the drug, because they affect normal cells in the body that naturally produce some of the target protein (although not in such high levels as the cancer cells). For example, a skin rash detected while on an EGFR inhibitor suggests the patient may be responding to the drug, because the drug targets the outer layer of the skin, where some EGFR is present on the surface of cells.

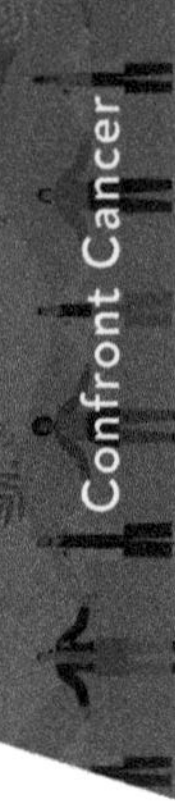

Now that we have looked at various treatments that may be available for your cancer, let's move on to how you might use your diagnostic information to choose the best therapy for yourself.

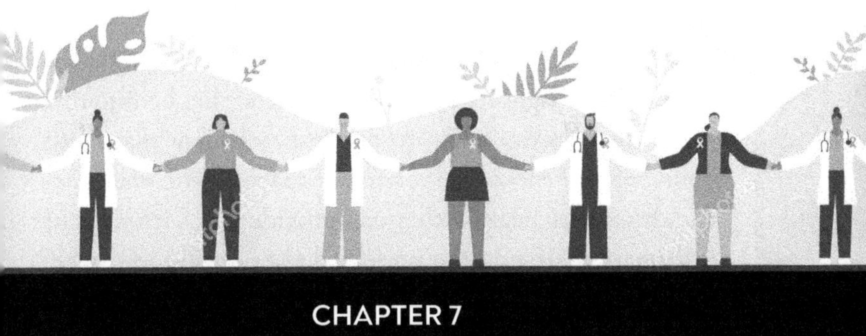

CHAPTER 7

USING YOUR DIAGNOSTIC INFORMATION TO INFORM TREATMENT OPTIONS

It bears repeating at this point: your diagnosis points to your treatment options. Think of your treatment options as a funnel. At the beginning, you know you have cancer of a specific organ which opens up many treatment options, including chemotherapy, targeted agents, and immunotherapy. Then you find out you have a certain subtype of that cancer, and the options become narrower. You may rule out certain types of treatment as they are better suited for other subtypes of cancer in that organ. Next, you find out you have (or don't have) specific genetic alterations in your tumor. This further narrows the choices until finally you are left with a limited number of options for treatment. Once you are at the bottom of the funnel, you need to ensure you know as much as you can about every treatment option open to you. That is the focus of this chapter.

Once you fully understand how your physician arrived at your cancer diagnosis and what confidence lies behind this diagnosis, you can begin to derive a treatment plan with your doctor. I encourage you to be proactive with your doctor about this, because they can provide you with a lot of information. The option presented to you will most likely have been derived using the clinical guidelines the doctor is following. In the United States, this is the National Comprehensive Cancer Network guidelines, and in the United Kingdom, it's the National Institute for Health and Care Excellence guidelines.

These guidelines provide the consensus and evidence-based opinion of a group of highly qualified and esteemed authors on the currently accepted approaches to treatment. Doctors who consult these guidelines are expected to use their independent medical judgment in individual clinical circumstances to determine any patient's care or management of treatment. There is separate guidance for every tumor type, and it usually comes as a flow chart showing which treatments a patient with a specific cancer diagnosis may benefit from. Your doctor can work through these guidelines with you.

Clinical cancer guidance is organized according to the anatomical location of your tumor and begins with the principles of diagnostic evaluation. This guidance suggests whether a biopsy should be performed based on specific features and, if so, which type of biopsy (discussed in Chapter 3). The features that doctors will use to make this evaluation include the size and location of the tumor, your medical history, and the availability of local hospital expertise. There will be one set of guidelines for the first treatment you should receive, then another set for which therapy you should have if the first one doesn't work, and so on. As you move through your treatments, you will have fewer options; you will have already encountered certain therapies, and in many circumstances, it won't make sense to have them again because your tumor is not likely to respond.

Doctors will monitor you regularly during each treatment to ensure the drugs you are taking are working and also to manage any side effects. If the tumor does not shrink, or you are not tolerating the therapy very well, they may give you an option during one of these monitoring visits to change your treatment. Your doctor will use the guidelines and knowledge of your previous experience and condition to determine a second treatment option. You may also have some more diagnostic testing done on either the biopsy already taken or a new biopsy. The purpose of more testing at this stage can be for two reasons:

1. The drug you were taking is known for causing a specific resistance pattern in the tumor. A new biopsy may show that this is the case, and then a very specific treatment option can be administered. For example, you may have lung cancer that was treated with an EGFR inhibitor that was initially working, but your recent

scans show that the tumor has started to grow again. You have another test that shows a new alteration in the EGFR gene is likely stopping your treatment from working. The next option is probably a different EGFR inhibitor that will work on cells with the new mutation.

2. There are several targeted options available to you, and the doctor would like to see whether you qualify for these options. For example, in the lung cancer case above, instead of a new EGFR mutation arising, you have developed resistance to the EGFR inhibitor by amplifying another gene called MET, so a MET inhibitor may be more appropriate.

CLINICAL TRIALS

After diagnosis, most of the treatments presented to you will have been fully tested in the clinic and approved by the overarching regulatory body, such as the FDA or the MHRA. Clinical trials are research studies that aim to evaluate a specific treatment or intervention that the regulatory bodies have not yet approved. They are used to find out whether a new treatment is safe and effective in people.

Doctors only perform a clinical trial when they think a new test or treatment is likely to improve the care and outcome of patients. Before starting a clinical trial, scientists evaluate the test or treatment in the laboratory. These types of research, termed *preclinical research*, may look at different aspects of the treatment to determine whether it is likely to be safe and effective on human tissue and organs. After preclinical research, treatment begins in people, and testing proceeds through a series of clinical trials to determine the treatment's safety and effectiveness. Before a clinical trial can begin, the background research and clinical plan must be submitted and approved by regulatory bodies to ensure it is as safe as possible for patients. When you are taking part in a clinical trial, doctors will closely monitor you to ensure the side effects are not too harsh and that the drug is performing effectively.

> *Doctors only perform a clinical trial when they think a new test or treatment is likely to improve the care and outcome of patients.*

Clinical trials have five phases; some treatments may not require them all.

PHASE 0 TRIALS

Phase 0 trials are the first clinical trials done on people. They aim to provide information to scientists and doctors about how human bodies process the drug and how they are affected by it. In these trials, doctors give a minimal dose of medicine to about ten or fifteen people. At this phase, the intention is not to treat sick people; therefore, these trials are often performed on healthy volunteers.

PHASE I TRIALS

Phase I trials aim to find the best dose for a new drug; that is, the dose that will be effective with the fewest side effects. Doctors test the medicine in a small group of around fifteen to thirty patients. The first few patients will receive a very low dose of the drug. Once the drug is considered safe at that dose, the next patients receive a slightly higher dose. This process is continued in a stepwise fashion with increasingly higher doses until side effects become too severe or the desired result is seen. In Phase I, the drug may help treat patients, but Phase I trials are primarily designed to test a drug's safety. If you are a patient in a Phase I trial and have received one of the very low doses, you may be permitted to change to a higher dose of treatment in order to gain more benefit from the drug once the higher doses are considered safe. These trials may also assess the safety of two drugs in combination.

You should bear in mind that being part of a Phase I clinical trial means you may be on a very low dose of a drug that is known to not have the desired effects on the tumor. You may also experience unexpected side effects in this phase.

If doctors determine the drug is safe enough for humans, testing continues to a Phase II clinical trial.

PHASE II TRIALS

Phase II trials aim to further assess the safety as well as the effectiveness of the drug. At this stage, doctors often test the drug among patients with a specific type of cancer or genetic alteration who are more likely to benefit from the drug. Phase II requires larger groups of patients than Phase I, and all patients are treated at the same dose, which is the recommended dose from the Phase I study. If a drug treats the patients effectively, the next step is generally a Phase III trial. Drugs that prove to be especially promising are sometimes approved after Phase II clinical trials, but Phase III clinical trials are often needed before regulatory bodies will approve the use of a new drug for the general public.

PHASE III TRIALS

Phase III trials compare a new drug against the current **standard of care** drug that is given to patients. These trials monitor the efficacy and side effects of both the standard of care drug and the investigational drug to assess which drug works better. Cancer clinical trials rarely use a placebo (fake pill) for the comparison, as it is not ethical to withhold treatment from a patient if there is a treatment option available.

Phase III trials are large and enroll one hundred or more patients. Often, Phase III trials are randomized, which means that the organizers randomly divide patients into two (or more) groups called *trial arms*. A computer program often assigns the groups. The simplest structure involves one group receiving the new treatment (the drug under investigation) while the other group receives the standard of care drug. Randomization is required to ensure that the people in both trial arms are similar and that the trial results are due to the treatment and not to other differences between the groups. You or your doctor cannot choose your group, and you may not even know which group you're in until the trial is over. Sometimes, you may already have received the drug being administered in the control arm, so it is essential to find out which drugs are used in each group before entering the trial.

As in the other phases, doctors closely monitor the patients, and the study will stop early if the new drug's side effects are too severe or if one group has much better results than the other.

If a drug passes the Phase III trials and is shown to be effective, it will be put forward for approval by the relevant regulatory bodies.

PHASE IV TRIALS

Phase IV trials test new drugs that regulatory bodies have approved. The drug is tested in hundreds or thousands of patients, allowing for more research on the side effects and safety of the drug. For example, it is necessary to test a large group of patients in order to discover rare side effects that appear in only a few individuals. Investigators can also learn more about how effective the drug is when used with other treatments.

CHOOSING WHETHER TO PARTICIPATE IN A TRIAL

Patients most frequently enter a clinical trial because they have very few treatment options, or when a particular investigational drug has been very promising in early phases and their doctor thinks they will gain more from the trial drug than from other options. When you're deciding whether to enter a clinical trial, it is essential to look at all this information to determine whether being part of a study is right for you. This includes finding out what your other options are.

When you are considering participating in a clinical trial, it is usually more important to understand the study's objective than what phase the trial is. A great place to find this information is by looking at prior research publications about the drug, including preclinical research and reports on the initial phases of the trial. These may be published online in peer-reviewed journals or in conference proceedings, such as those of the American Society of Clinical Oncology and American Association for Cancer Research. Two good places to look for this kind of information are PubMed and Google Scholar. Some of the scientific details you find are likely to be complex; if you have trouble interpreting them, bring the information to your doctor, who can explain it to you. If you are in one of the later phases of the trial, it may be possible to find out what side effects patients experienced while on the drug in previous phases and whether the research team saw that the drug showed any benefit to patients. These details are also often reported in peer-reviewed journals and conference proceedings.

A clear understanding of what will be expected of you before and during the trial will help you decide how participating in the study will affect your life. The nature of a clinical trial means doctors will monitor you closely, which brings the advantage that you will have more support from your cancer care team. On the flip side, the additional monitoring means you will have to attend more appointments, sometimes when you're not feeling your best. You will have more tests, which may mean you will have to have more blood taken, or you may have to be admitted to the hospital for a few days. Before entering the clinical trial, ask about what kind of treatment you will have and how often you will have to take it. Find out what testing they will require you to have, how often, and where you will need to go to have these tests.

Compare the clinical trial drug against other options in terms of likely effectiveness and side effects. Ask your doctor if there are any other risks that the investigational treatment may pose compared to the drug considered standard of care. Here are some more questions to consider:

- How will you know if the drug is working? In most cases, the measure of whether a drug is working on a clinical trial is very similar to that of the standard of care drug—you will have regular scans of your tumor to see whether its size has decreased. Before entering the trial, you can ask how often these scans will take place, whether you will have access to the results, who will pay for them, and what they will entail.

- How often will you have to go to the hospital or clinic? You may need to be admitted into the hospital for a particular test or treatment as part of the trial. If this is the case, find out how often you will have to do this and for how long.
- Who will pay for the extra hospital or clinic visits? In some cases, the sponsor running the trial may pay for these expenses. In other cases, your insurance may cover the treatment.
- How long will the clinical trial last, and how long are you likely to be a part of it? The length of the clinical trial is important information to have. You can get this information by looking at how long patients in previous clinical trial phases were on the treatment.
- Is there a likelihood you may stop treatment earlier than expected and, if so, why? Find out whether doctors removed any people from the clinical trials in previous phases and why they were removed.
- Will there be any additional genetic or other testing involved? The extensive patient monitoring

in a clinical trial often extends to more genetic testing of your tumor, either via new biopsies or using what remains from previous biopsies. These additional tests may uncover information that could open future treatment options to you. Many clinical trials will perform genetic studies on your tumor before and during treatment to see how your tumor changes during treatment. You may have access to these results.

- What will happen when the trial has finished? Is long-term follow-up care part of the trial? What would this involve? If the treatment has been working, can you keep taking this drug after the clinical trial ends? If you were on a Phase I clinical trial where doctors treat patients at different doses and you received a lower dose, can you get the higher dose once it is considered safe?

Most of this information can be obtained from your doctor (or your doctor can help you find it), but it may be possible to contact other people on the trial or those who have been on a similar trial. A discussion with one of these patients may bring aspects of the trial to light that you hadn't previously considered.

Choosing to be part of a clinical trial is a big decision. You may find it helpful to include friends and family members in your research and decision-making process to ensure you are taking the right path for yourself. You can also get a second opinion from another doctor to help you with this process.

If you decide to participate in the clinical trial, they will ask you to sign a consent form. This form contains valuable information about the trial and what your participation in the trial may entail. You can ask the doctor for a copy of the consent form to aid in your information gathering.

BENEFITS OF PARTICIPATION

Every clinical trial has its unique benefits and risks, but here are some potential benefits of taking part in a clinical trial:

- You are helping others. You might help others who get the same disease in the future by helping to advance cancer research.
- You have more treatment options. You may get a treatment that is not available outside of the trial, and it may either work better or be safer than the standard of care.
- You have more control. A clinical trial may open up treatment options where you had few or no options before. As such, this provides you with a level of control over the management of your treatment.
- You have more support. Because of the extensive monitoring in a clinical trial, you will go to

the hospital and clinic to see your cancer care team more often than you would on a non-investigative treatment. This monitoring means doctors can detect potential issues earlier than they would during standard of care treatment.

- There may be a financial benefit. The center running the trial may pay for part or all of your care and expenses during the trial.

RISKS ASSOCIATED WITH PARTICIPATION

Agreeing to participate in trials of unlicensed medications or other treatments is not without hazards, although the researchers and clinicians running the trial will have undertaken risk assessments and received approval from the authorities, ensuring that the risk to individual participants is minimized. The following are general risks for participating in a clinical trial:

- The outcome of the treatment is unknown for the population. The treatment under investigation may have unknown side effects or risks. These could be worse or better than those associated with standard therapies.

- The outcome of the treatment is unknown for you. Every treatment works differently in different people. There is some knowledge of how people respond to standard of care treatments, but this knowledge is minimal in clinical trials, especially in early phases. The new treatment may benefit some people, but not everyone.

- Participation will require more effort. The extensive monitoring on a clinical trial means you may need to visit the clinic more often for tests.

- There are more unknowns. If the clinical trial is randomized, you may not be able to choose which treatment you receive, and if the study is *blinded*, you (and likely your doctor) will not know which treatment you are being given.

There may be administrative differences. Insurers cover the costs of standard of care drugs but may not cover all costs of the clinical trial, so it is critical to know who will pay for your care. Often the clinical trial sponsor will pay for some aspects of your care, but maybe not all. Note that Medicare usually covers clinical trial costs. Contact your insurance provider and ask your doctor about this.

Weigh the general and specific risks for a particular trial against your other options with the potential benefits of taking part in the trial. Be clear about why you want to participate in the trial and what the best and worst scenarios may be.

GOVERNING BODIES IN CLINICAL TRIALS

To ensure that research teams perform clinical trials correctly and in the best interests of patients, several governing bodies assess and inspect clinical trials. I will only discuss here the governing bodies that are involved in clinical trials in the United States; similar bodies handle clinical trials in other countries.

The study sponsor takes responsibility for and initiates a clinical investigation. The sponsor can be an individual or a pharmaceutical/biotechnology company, academic institution, private organization, or other organization.

The principal investigator is a medically trained professional whose primary responsibility is to ensure patient safety in the clinical trial. This person is required to inform the study sponsor immediately if severe side effects occur.

The institutional review board (IRB) is a group that meets regularly to ensure that the trial organizers are conducting the clinical trial according to federal laws. To set up a clinical trial, researchers must send a clinical trial protocol (a detailed plan describing the trial) to the IRB. The IRB decides whether the study will look to answer a worthwhile question and considers the safety of participants. Trial organizers send a patient consent form to the IRB for review, and the IRB ensures that this form is accurate, complete, and easy to understand. Once a clinical trial starts, the IRB will monitor it to identify problems. If you are a participant in a clinical trial, you can contact the IRB with questions you may have.

The Office for Human Research Protections is the government's principal agency for protecting people's safety in clinical trials. This office ensures that organizers follow the rules stated in the informed consent and protocols; it can stop a clinical trial if it finds problems.

The US Food and Drug Administration (FDA) approves drugs to be given to patients. Once a Phase II or III clinical trial is complete, the FDA reviews the results and decides whether the new treatment is safe and effective. Before the start of a clinical trial, researchers must gain approval from the FDA to begin. The FDA inspects hospitals and laboratories performing the work for clinical trials to ensure they follow the correct procedures. If the FDA finds problems, it can prevent a hospital or doctor from continuing the trial.

HOW TO FIND A CLINICAL TRIAL

Often, your doctor will let you know of a clinical trial they think may be suitable for you or that they are conducting themselves. However, new clinical trials emerge all the time, and your doctor can't know about all of them, so be proactive. You can look for clinical trials online or in other places to identify more options for treatment.

The search results you find on clinical trial websites include information such as

- a description of each study
- factors that people must meet to be a part of the trial (inclusion and exclusion criteria)

- the name of a contact person

These websites help you focus your search using specific terms for your type and stage of cancer, the treatment you're looking for—be it chemotherapy, immunotherapy, or targeted therapy—and how far you are willing to travel.

ClinicalTrials.gov is a fantastic website providing free access to information on current publicly and privately supported clinical trials for a wide range of diseases and conditions (not just cancer). The National Institutes of Health in the United States developed and maintains the website, which includes information on clinical trials from all fifty states and 219 countries. The sponsor or principal investigator of the clinical study provides and maintains the entry for their trial.

Clinical trials are registered on ClinicalTrials.gov when they begin, and sponsors provide updates throughout the study. Often, the results of the study are also submitted once the trial ends. The entry for a clinical trial contains the following information:

- disease or cancer type under study;
- intervention, drug, or regimen under study;
- title, description, and design of the study;
- requirements the patient must meet to be eligible for the study;
- locations of the study;

- contact information for each study location;
- links to relevant information on other health websites, such as patient health information and scientific studies.

Some records also include further information on the study, such as

- the number of participants starting and completing the study (along with their age and gender);
- the outcomes of the study; and
- the summary of side effects experienced by study participants.

You can use this site to find clinical trials that you may be eligible to participate in and where doctors are conducting them. You can also look up any clinical trials that your doctor has suggested and find more information about them. I suggest you set up an initial search for your specific cancer type with a location boundary; this will show you results for trials taking place in locations to which you are willing to travel.

The critical information that you need to pull from each trial is

- the phase of the clinical trial (found under Study Design on the study page);
- whether the study is currently recruiting (found in the top right green box of the study page);

- the closest study site to you (found under Contacts and Locations toward the bottom of the study page);
- the intervention model of the trial—for example, whether it is randomized or not (found under Study Design); and
- the inclusion and exclusion criteria, which are required to determine the eligibility of individuals (found under the Eligibility Criteria section).

You can check the inclusion and exclusion criteria yourself to see whether you would be eligible for a trial. Sometimes you will need more information than you have at hand, in which case, you can request help from your health care team. You can produce a spreadsheet with a short list of the clinical trials you are interested in and information on the key points above. Take this to the next appointment to discuss with your doctor.

Once you have a list of clinical trials that you think you may be eligible for, it can still be challenging to determine which ones are best suited for you. In addition to your primary care doctor and cancer doctor, talk with as many relevant people as you can about the specific trials. These people could be the principal investigator on the trial (a doctor) or a research coordinator (usually a nurse). A research coordinator can serve as a link between you and the doctor and will provide eligibility information. As with all these decisions, finding a second opinion from another cancer doctor is wise, especially if you can find one with expertise in the specific trial or with the type of cancer you have. Finally, talk to your support group—your family members and friends. While the final decision is yours, their insight may make you think about aspects of the trials you hadn't previously considered.

STATISTICS ASSOCIATED WITH YOUR TREATMENT

One of the first questions people diagnosed with cancer often ask is, "What's the chance of survival?" or, "How long do I have?" Your doctor may use statistics to help you understand this. Statistics are estimates that describe trends in large numbers of people. You can use these numbers to evaluate treatment options and compare your likely outcome on each treatment. What statistics cannot do is predict how well the treatment will work for you individually; everyone is different, and your response to treatment may differ from the average response in a large group.

The following explains some of the jargon your doctor may use in explaining statistics to you.

DISEASE-ASSOCIATED STATISTICS

Prognosis is the likely outcome or chance of recovery. Doctors may refer to an individual person's prognosis (their particular likely outcome) or the prognosis of a large group (the general outcomes seen in people with cancer like yours).

The **overall survival** rate is the percentage of people alive after a certain time has passed from diagnosis. The time length used can vary, but cancer statistics are often represented as a five-year survival rate.

The five-year relative survival rate is the percentage of people alive five years after diagnosis, not including deaths from other causes. For example, the five-year relative survival rate for women with breast cancer is about 90 percent, which means that about ninety out of every one hundred women with breast cancer will be alive five years after their diagnosis.

Survival rates can also be specific to cancer stages. For instance, the five-year relative survival rate for breast cancer with distant metastases (in which secondary tumors are present at distant locations in the body) is 28 percent. This means that twenty-eight out of every one hundred women that have breast cancer with distant metastases will be alive five years after diagnosis.

Scientists can only generate these statistics by looking back over the past five years and finding out how many people with a particular type of cancer have survived. Because of this, some statistics may not reflect newer therapies that became available during the prior five years, so these values are usually at the lower end of the current survival rate.

TREATMENT-ASSOCIATED STATISTICS

Disease-free survival rate is the percentage of people who have no signs or symptoms of cancer (also referred to as **complete remission**) after completion of treatment.

Progression-free survival rate is the percentage of people who have no tumor growth or cancer spread during or after treatment, which means the cancer is still there but is not growing or spreading.

How can you use survival statistics to compare treatment options?

Compare the potential outcomes of your different treatment options by looking at their five-year survival rates. These statistics will allow you to assess the likelihood of you responding to treatment and the possibility that the treatment will extend your life. Weigh these outcomes against other factors, such as potential side effects, to make an informed decision.

DECISION-MAKING CHECKLIST FOR TREATMENT

To make an informed decision on which treatment option to take, whether or not it includes a clinical trial, you can use the following checklist.

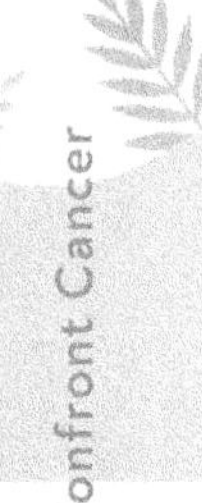
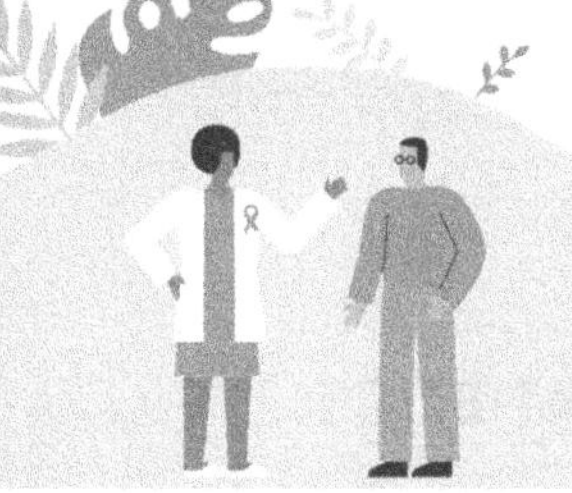
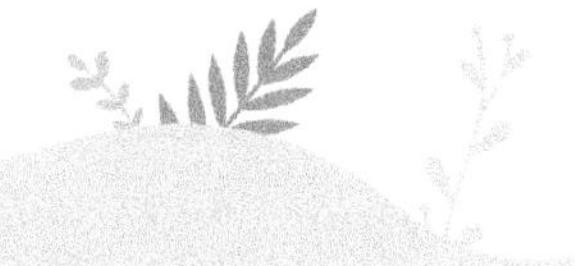

1

Understand the diagnosis.

- How confident is my doctor that this diagnosis is accurate?

- What information led to the diagnosis?

- Do all the tests (the scans, pathology, and genetics) point to the same diagnosis?

- If there is doubt, are there further tests I can have to confirm the diagnosis?

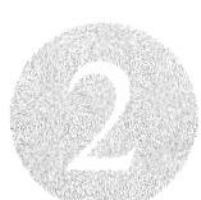

Know the options.

- Given my diagnosis, what treatment options do I have?

- Which options are considered standard of care?

- What clinical trials could I join?

- What are the expected end points of each treatment (e.g., a cure, longer life, or better quality of life)?

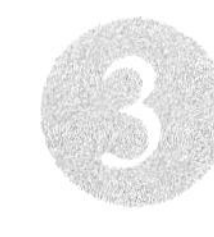

Understand the goals of treatment.

- o How and when will I know if my treatment is working?

- o Is the goal to shrink the tumor or alleviate symptoms?

- o What can I expect as outcomes of the treatment?

- o What would be the next step if this didn't work?

Ask about the side effects of each treatment option.

- O What side effects can I expect in both the short-term and the long-term?

- O How severe will they be?

- O Will they stop me from leading a normal life?

- O Will I still be able to work?

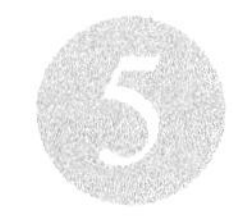

Consider the risks and benefits of each treatment option.

- O How likely is it that this treatment will work (overall survival, progression-free survival)?

- O What will my quality of life be like while on this treatment?

- O How often will I have to go to the hospital?

- O Can I take the treatment by mouth, or does it need to be injected?

6

Get a second (and even third) opinion.

- O Does another doctor with experience with my cancer have the same opinion?

Research the costs of the treatments.

- O What are the expenses related to treatment options?

- O Does my insurance cover the costs?

- O Do I need to find financial support services available to people living with cancer?

- O If I cannot work during the treatment, how will that affect me?

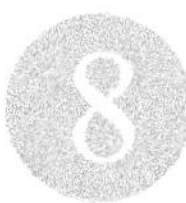

Discuss with friends and family.

- O Who can I trust to discuss these options with me?

Having gathered all this information, you may find yourself still stuck deciding which option to choose. You can start by weighing the pros and cons of each treatment. Make a table with all the questions above as rows and a column for each treatment option. Put a score in each box between 1 and 3 (1 = good, 3 = bad) for each question. Then add up all the rows for each column. Which column has the lowest score based on these questions?

You can also assign a weight for each question to signify how important it is to you. For example, many people may be most concerned with how well the treatment will work, and so this factor could have a higher weight. If that is the case, assign that row a weight of two and the others a weight of one; then multiply the "how well will a treatment work" scores by two before calculating the column totals. Assigning these weights personalizes the decision, but you could also add a row for "how do I feel about this treatment?" This decision-making strategy can be helpful if you have strong opinions about a specific drug because of side effects, experiences your family or friends have shared, or any other reason.

You are at the bottom of the funnel now, but by working through this chapter, you should have uncovered all the options available to you and your unique situation. The next chapter summarizes the whole process and offers some advice on how to make the best decision.

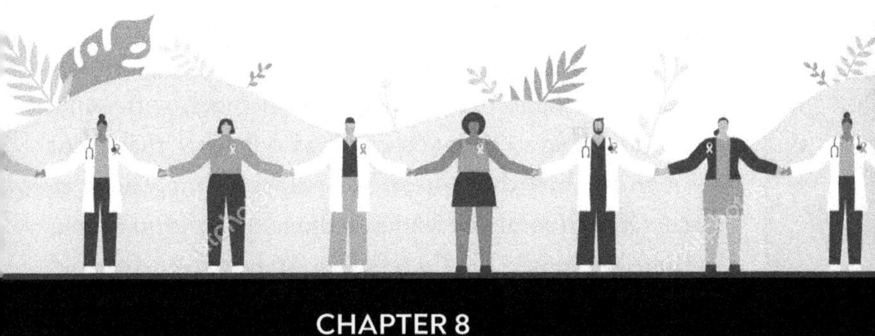

CHAPTER 8

FORMING A PLAN

Everyone is unique. Provided with the same information, different people will prefer different options. This chapter collates all the previous chapters to build on the knowledge you have gained, check that you have completed every step, and help you make an informed decision.

The focus of this book is to help you with information gathering to understand your diagnosis and identify your treatment options. However, you should not forget a third and crucial step: developing a support network. One thing you can be sure of in your situation is that you are not alone; 1.8 million new cancer cases are diagnosed each year in the United States. You are one of many people

you should not forget a third and crucial step: developing a support network.

who have navigated a similar diagnosis. There are many resources available that can put you in touch with some of these people so that you can find out what they went through and how they coped. Sometimes it simply helps to discuss it with someone who is in the same position as you. In the 2014 movie *The Fault in Our Stars*, sixteen-year-old Hazel struggled to find people she could relate to, especially when she was dealing with some difficult side effects. Making these connections early on can help you make decisions now as well as navigate other issues later on. You can also use your existing support network of friends and family to help you gather information, ask questions, and discuss the best steps forward.

Now let's lay out a plan to find out which treatment is best for you.

TAKE TIME TO PROCESS

When you first receive a cancer diagnosis, the new world you have been launched into can seem daunting. Take some time to let the news sink in. Having this time to process the situation will allow you to think about what is important to you, which will be useful for making informed decisions later. During this time, your health care team will indicate how quickly you need to act. If you have a slow-growing type of tumor, you may have lots of time, but if you have a more aggressive cancer, time may be of the essence. Your health care team may be planning urgent tests, surgeries, and treatments to get you started with your cancer management straight away. You can use this information to determine how long you can take to process the news.

Ironically, a cancer diagnosis is often life affirming, and your priorities may dramatically change during this time. In time, you may come to feel gratitude for the gifts of awareness gained because of your diagnosis.

RESEARCH YOUR HEALTH CARE TEAM

After you have taken time to process, spend some time researching the doctor you were referred to for your treatment. Use the internet to learn about their background and determine how much experience they have with your specific cancer. Identify whether they have any research commitments that could influence the treatments they may offer you.

For example, if your doctor has presented at scientific conferences about your specific cancer, you know they are experienced in that field. What were the titles of those presentations? Was the doctor reporting on clinical trials or new treatments from their own lab?

Find out whether your doctor has received any advanced or specialized training. Confirm that they are board certified in oncology. The following societies provide databases to search for your doctor to find out if they are board certified:

- The American Society of Clinical Oncology
- The American Board of Medical Specialties
- The American Medical Association
- The American College of Surgeons

In addition, Medicare.gov offers a searchable database of doctors who accept Medicare.

Depending on your eventual treatment plan, you may need a medical, surgical, and radiation oncologist. A medical oncologist treats cancer using drugs, such as conventional chemotherapy, targeted therapy, and immunotherapy. A surgical oncologist removes the tumor and nearby tissue during surgery, and also may be the one who takes a biopsy for your diagnosis. A radiation oncologist treats cancer using radiation therapy.

Check that your doctor participates in your health insurance plan. Often you can look up doctors and associated details about them on your health insurance website. You can also ask the doctor's office staff which insurance plans they accept.

You need to feel comfortable talking with your doctor and health care team, so arrange to meet them either in the office or via a virtual meeting. Find out whether they speak in a way you understand and check that they provide answers to your questions. Ask the doctor about their credentials and experience:

- When did they get their medical degree and how long have they practiced medicine?
- How many patients with this type of cancer do they treat per year?
- Do they have access to clinical trials and, if so, which ones?
- Where would you receive your treatment—at the office or elsewhere?
- Where are the laboratories that would perform your pathology and genomic tests—on-site or elsewhere?
- Would you be able to speak to the pathologist to ask questions?
- Does the doctor use large genomic sequencing panels for diagnosis?
- Can you reach your doctor and health care team in the evening, on the weekend, or on holidays?

It is also helpful to find out about the extended health care team that will provide your care if you decide to use that doctor. Does the office have support staff (registered nurses, social workers, nutrition specialists, pharmacists, counselors)? Ask how they would be involved in your care. You may require specialized care through your treatment, and you can ask specifically about access to those professionals, including genetic counselors, doctors or nurses specialized in pain management, radiologists (doctors who interpret imaging tests and scans), and rehabilitation therapists (e.g., physical, occupational, speech, or recreational therapists). Some professionals can help with your general well-being, such as mental health professionals and spiritual advisers.

Here are other questions you can ask about the health care team:

- Is there a person on the health care team who would be your primary contact (these people are often called *patient educators* or *patient navigators)?*
- Who would that be, and when will they be available?
- Are you able to speak with them comfortably?
- What can this person help you with in terms of support?

Once you have gathered this information about the doctor you have been referred to, you can begin looking for other doctors who may be more suitable. Start by looking within a certain geographical distance on your health insurance website, and narrow it down to the doctors who have experience in your type of cancer. Set up meetings with them, either in person or virtually, to ask the same questions you did of your own doctor. Remember, you may not ultimately use this doctor, but you could go to them in the future for a second opinion. Most insurance plans will pay for a second opinion, and so it can be helpful even at this stage to identify other doctors who have relevant experience and are covered by your insurance.

You may identify a doctor with a lot of experience, but their team does not have everything you are looking for. This doctor would be an excellent candidate for a potential second opinion. Be mindful, too, that you may need a second opinion on several aspects of your cancer, such as diagnosis or staging, interpretation of scans and lab reports, identification of clinical trials, or formulation of treatment plans.

FORMULATE A TESTING AND TREATMENT PLAN

Once you have decided who will be your primary cancer doctor and you have a short list of candidates for a second opinion, start to discuss the plan for determining your diagnosis.

To illustrate the importance of having these discussions at this early stage, let's consider an example case study.

A sixty-year-old man, a non-smoker who had been coughing for two months, went to the doctor. The doctor referred him for a CT scan, which showed he had a lung tumor that had reached some of his lymph nodes (remember: the lymph nodes are the bean-like organs that drain your tissues). A CT-guided core needle biopsy of the lung tumor and lymph node revealed **grade** 3 lung adenocarcinoma by examination under the microscope. An MRI scan showed a small tumor in his head, suggesting the tumor had already spread. Comprehensive genetic testing showed negative tests for the three most prominent genetic alterations associated with lung cancer. However, a rare genetic alteration called an NTRK fusion was detected. NTRK fusions are where part of the NTRK protein becomes fused to another protein, and they are found in 0.1–3 percent of all lung cancers. Most patients who don't have a comprehensive genomic test only have targeted testing of the three genes that most often have alterations in lung cancer. If this man had only targeted testing, his treatment options would be limited, as all the markers would be negative, indicating that targeted treatments would not work. In this case, the patient would probably be treated with conventional chemotherapy and immunotherapy—a regimen with considerable side effects, where the average time before the tumor starts growing again is approximately 8.8 months. Luckily, the comprehensive genomic testing showed a rare NTRK fusion, suggesting the tumor may respond to an NTRK inhibitor. He went on a treatment course of larotrectinib (an NTRK inhibitor) and experienced only minimal side effects. A scan at two months showed the tumors had not significantly changed, and so he continued treatment. A scan at eighteen months showed the tumors had both shrunk! This man was still doing well eighteen months after diagnosis and continued the treatment. He would likely have stopped the other treatments well before this point, and the tumors would have started growing again. As the alternative regimen would have included aggressive chemotherapy, he would have experienced more significant side effects, such as losing his hair and feeling very unwell. For this man, identifying a NTRK fusion meant eighteen months of good-quality life with the hope of more.

For this man, identifying a NTRK fusion meant eighteen months of good-quality life with the hope of more.

This is why I urge you to speak with your doctor about comprehensive genomic testing at the outset. If they are not suggesting it, why not? If you feel it may be too expensive, you can discuss with your insurance provider whether it would be covered. If the results will take too long, find out how long, and ask what can be done while you wait for the results. If the biopsy you are having will not yield enough material for all the tests, ask about a different biopsy, or suggest you have a genomic test from blood instead. Do whatever you can to get the maximum possible information about your tumor.

"Comprehensive" genomic tests can vary widely. Some may include twenty genes; others may have five hundred. Find out which one is proposed for you, and which ones your insurance will cover. The tests with fewer genes generally require less tissue but also provide less information.

After you have had the biopsy and tests, ask your doctor for the reports. Each report will state the genes included in the test, any mutations that were found, and their interpretations. If the results were inconclusive, ask your doctor for more details. Record this meeting with your doctor, so that you can return to it later, as you may not immediately understand or take in everything your doctor says. Ask your doctor whether you or they can speak to the person who wrote the report if you need clarification. If a test failed or the result was inconclusive, is there time and enough tissue to rerun it?

Once you are happy with the test results, discuss the final diagnosis with your doctor. Ask how they arrived at the diagnosis. Did all tests point to this diagnosis, or is there any discrepancy between tests? If there is a likelihood your tumor could fall into two different diagnostic categories, what are they, and do they have different treatment options?

Once you have a clear diagnosis, begin to discuss what your options are. What are the treatment plans for this diagnosis? What are the risks? Use Chapter 6 to help you.

CONSIDER A SECOND OPINION

Once you have a diagnosis from your primary cancer doctor, now is the best time to get a second opinion. Consider how long it will take to get this opinion and how vital it is to get started on your first treatment. Then, if you decide to go ahead, email them all the test and scan reports (ideally containing the scan images) in advance so they can get a handle on your case before you discuss anything further. At the appointment, do not provide any of the interpretation from your primary cancer doctor (although the doctor may have seen it anyway); let them come to their own conclusion as to what your diagnosis and treatment plan should be. This doctor may suggest ordering more tests, in which case you may need to ensure that the leftover specimen is made available to them.

As with your primary cancer doctor, record the meeting so that you can return to the conversation as questions arise in your mind afterward. Ask the same questions to clarify how the doctor has arrived at their diagnosis and why they propose the particular treatment plan. If they give you the same diagnosis as the first doctor, and both doctors agree that the diagnosis was soundly based on the investigational findings, you can rest easy that you have a solid diagnosis and can proceed to devise your treatment plan.

If the second doctor gives you a different diagnosis than the first, now is the time to share the earlier diagnosis with the second doctor and discuss why the two may differ. It may be that the tests are contradictory or one was inconclusive, and the doctors have interpreted them differently. How can you clear up this discrepancy? Are there more tests that could be ordered? Would repeating the original tests help? It may be that the second doctor ordered more tests and based their diagnosis on this new information; in this case, take the fresh information to your primary cancer doctor to see whether it changes their diagnosis.

If you cannot clear up the discrepancy based on these methods, consider a third (and maybe even a fourth) opinion to gain a consensus on diagnosis.

Once you have arrived at a diagnosis, you can begin to discuss your treatment plan. Depending on your diagnosis, you may have several options to consider. Get as much information about these options as you can from each doctor you consulted.

> *Don't just trust the treatment options the doctors have provided. Bring more opportunities to the table!*

Don't just trust the treatment options the doctors have provided. Bring more opportunities to the table! There may be newer options that your doctor is not yet aware of. These could be newly approved drugs or clinical trials. See Chapter 7 for how to research these options. Bring the information in, speak to your doctor about it, and ask the appropriate questions.

MAKE A DECISION THAT'S RIGHT FOR YOU

Your doctor can provide you with information on the treatment goals, but make sure you think about your desired outcomes for the treatment and beyond. Everyone's values are different, and you want to make sure this decision is right for you. You can listen to the information and advice given by your health care team, family, and friends, but this is ultimately your decision. Some people may be willing to undergo high-risk surgery if it is likely to cure their cancer, while others would be more willing to endure the pain from a different treatment in order to avoid surgery. The key is to identify the option that best fits your desired outcome.

Once you think you have decided, write down what you expect from this option in terms of how the treatment will go and what the outcome will be. Then use these expectations to run through your thoughts with your doctor and find out whether they are reasonable. This process will ensure you have correctly interpreted all the information your doctors have given you and any additional information you have gathered independently.

When your doctor considers the expectations that you have laid out for them and the information on which they are based, they can fill in any holes that might be missing. They can also correct any wrong assumptions. In particular, ensure you have the correct assumptions about side effects, cost, pain, and recovery time for the choice you have made.

After this appointment, re-evaluate your decision. Does it still make sense to you? Don't feel as though you're unable to change your mind at this point. Making these decisions is rarely easy. You may iterate through this process several times before you finally settle on the choice that makes the most sense for your diagnosis and situation.

PREPARE FOR YOUR TREATMENT

Once you have decided on the course of action, make plans to ensure you can do your part to get the best outcome possible while minimizing side effects and pain and maximizing your quality of life. For example, while you are undergoing treatment, what is the best diet for you? How much and which type of exercise should you do? Answers to these questions may evolve as you go through your treatment. Every time you see your doctor, more information will be available on how you are doing, so you should ask whether you need to adjust your plan along the way.

Finally, share your decision with your loved ones. Once you have shared your diagnosis with them, they will be keen to know what is planned and how they can help. You can set up processes at this stage so that you don't have to individually call, text, or email large numbers of concerned friends and family members.

- Make a new voice mail message every day, or when something changes.

- Post online. Several free sites allow you to post your progress along with pictures. Examples include Caring Bridge and Lotsa Helping Hands.
- Delegate this task to a close loved one.

You may also want to discuss your decision with an attorney. They can advise you on any legal documents that can be prepared, such as a will, power of attorney, or a do-not-resuscitate (DNR) order. These documents will ensure your decisions are put in writing and will be adhered to in the future.

Once you have your decision and action plan based on a sound diagnosis, you can confidently move forward. Remember how you felt when you first got the diagnosis? How do you feel now? Hopefully, you have a sense that you are more in control, with a better understanding of your particular situation. However, the process of your active involvement in your treatment decision does not end here. You should continually discuss how you are doing with your health care team, checking in with them to assess whether the plan is progressing as you and they expected.

> *Just because your friend or neighbor had a similar type of cancer and got a certain treatment doesn't mean that will be the right option for you.*

To reiterate: everyone is unique. Provided with the same information, different people will prefer different options. Just because your friend or neighbor had a similar type of cancer and got a certain treatment doesn't mean that will be the right option for you. Dig deep and find out what is best for you. Your future self will thank you.

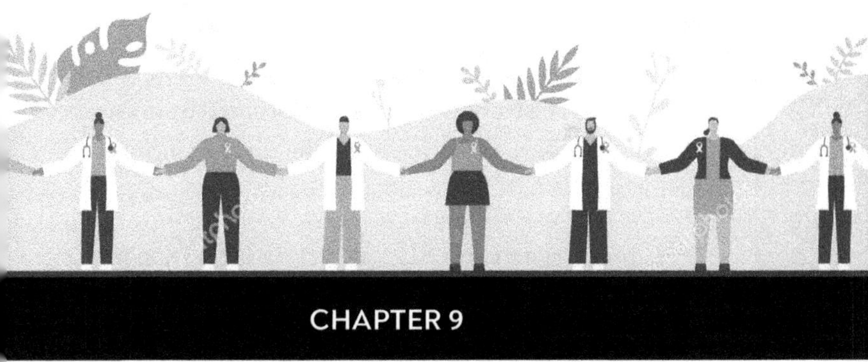

CHAPTER 9

WHAT IF THE CANCER RETURNS?

Treatment of cancer can be a multistage process. It may or may not have been your doctor's expectation that the first treatment plan would cure you. Or you may have come off your first treatment with a favorable outcome, but the tumor has come back several months or even years later. If this happens, don't despair; you still have all the tools you learned in this book, and this chapter will guide you through what may be different this time.

When you had your first treatment, most of the cancer cells were killed off, but a few cancer cells that were undetectable to current testing methods may have remained in your body. Those cells could have lain dormant for a while, but eventually they multiplied, resulting in a detectable level of cancer cells. When this happens, it is called a **relapse** or **recurrence**.

The newly detectable cancer cells may be in a similar place to where your cancer originated or they could be in another part of your body. Recurrence can be divided into the following types

- **local recurrence:** The cancer cells are seen in the same place where the cancer originated, and there has been no spread to other parts of the body.
- **regional recurrence:** The cancer cells have spread to the lymph nodes and surrounding tissue in the area of your original cancer.
- **distant recurrence:** The cancer cells have spread to other areas of your body from where your cancer was first located. Some cancer types will commonly recur in specific organs.

The word *cure* is not perfectly applicable to cancer. The health care field considers some cancers cured when they are undetectable five years after diagnosis, but relapse after five years is still a slight possibility.

In very rare cases, it could be that this emerging cancer is new and completely unrelated to the first one, but usually the detection of cancer cells will mean that cells from the original cancer have multiplied to detectable levels again.

At this point, it may seem like hope is lost, but this time, it will be easier for you to navigate. You know more about your cancer and about the procedures you may have to undergo, you have more connections, and you've done it all before. You already have your list of doctors for second and third opinions.

After your last round of treatment, your doctor probably gave you a schedule of monitoring checkups to test whether the cancer has returned. You were also probably told to watch out for signs and symptoms that might indicate a recurrence. It is important to watch out for these because, for most forms of cancer, a local recurrence may still be curable. However, if you wait too long and the cancer has time to spread to other parts of the body, the likelihood of a cure diminishes. Even when a cure isn't possible, there are treatments that can shrink the tumor and slow the cancer cells' growth, which can reduce your pain and other symptoms and may help you live longer.

Before looking at the next treatment step, think about whether now may be an appropriate time for a break. If you have had a long and arduous treatment path since your diagnosis, pausing may help you gain some strength and clarity before your next treatment. It can give you time to focus again on what is important in your life, which may influence your decisions for the next treatment. In some cases, it may not be wise to take a break from treatment, but it is worth speaking to your health care team about it if you feel it would be helpful.

All the steps outlined in Chapter 8 should be considered again with no omissions. Why must I have all the tests again, you may ask? Simply put, your cancer may have changed. Consider back to Chapter 2, where we discussed that different parts of your cancer could have unique attributes. Think of the cells in your tumor as a variety of grapes in a bowl—some are red, some are green, some have seeds, and others don't. There is a treatment you can apply that will make the seeds explode. This treatment causes the grapes with the seeds to burst, leaving mainly the seedless grapes. Some of the grapes with seeds adapt a protection mechanism by developing a thick, wrinkly skin a bit like a raisin. As a consequence, even though the seeds exploded in these raisin-like grapes, they still survive. Now the grapes look different—there are some raisin-like grapes in the bowl. If similar changes within your tumor happened during your first treatment, you need to know about it. You may be given the option at this stage to have Treatment A or Treatment B. Maybe those raisin-like grapes would be resistant to Treatment A because of their thick skin, but they could be sensitive to Treatment B. You can find out about new changes that have occurred in your cancer by having another biopsy or a genetic test. These changes are more likely to have happened if your first treatment appeared to work very well and then stopped working, or if your first treatment removed all evidence of the tumor and then it came back after some time.

In addition to the changes that occurred in your tumor, you may also have experienced considerable changes in your body and mental health. You may be weaker, mentally and physically; or you may be stronger and more determined to beat this. Your opinion on the potential side effects may have changed based on how well or poorly you tolerated the last treatment. You may not want to travel long distances now or spend long periods in the hospital. You may now have a better support circle, including health care providers and other people going through similar times. Reflecting on what has changed can help you make the next decision.

After your first treatment, you may have more information about your cancer and general health based on how you responded. Were you less able to tolerate the therapy than you expected? Did your cancer react in the way the doctors expected? Have they found new tumors elsewhere, or has the tumor spread further into the tissue? In addition, more information about your type of cancer may have come out of research studies and been presented at conferences or in scientific journals since you researched your original treatment. New treatments and clinical trials may even be available.

The treatments for recurrence will likely differ from the treatments you were offered the first time. This is because you have already had the other treatments, and the cancer cells that remain in your body survived those, so it is unlikely they will work this time. However, there are still clinical guidelines (see the National Comprehensive Cancer Network guidelines in the Useful Links section) that are followed at recurrence, and you and your care team can consult them to define the options. Options at this stage are going to be more limited than those the first time around, and so you may have to consider clinical trials this time even if you were not keen to take those risks before.

An important part of assessing your treatment options is finding out the likely outcomes using statistics, as we discussed in Chapter 7. The outcomes of a recurrence are different (and worse) than those at first diagnosis, so make sure the numbers you look at are for recurrent or metastatic cancer.

As always, a critical step in this process is the need for a second opinion. Another doctor may prefer you to stay on (or go back on) the first treatment you had, or may suggest new trials for which you have now become eligible.

Embarking on a second treatment for your cancer after finding out it has come back can feel crushing, but remember: you have all the tools you have learned in this book and many connections to help you with the decision. You have done it before. You know what is best for you. Use all this experience to plan your next steps.

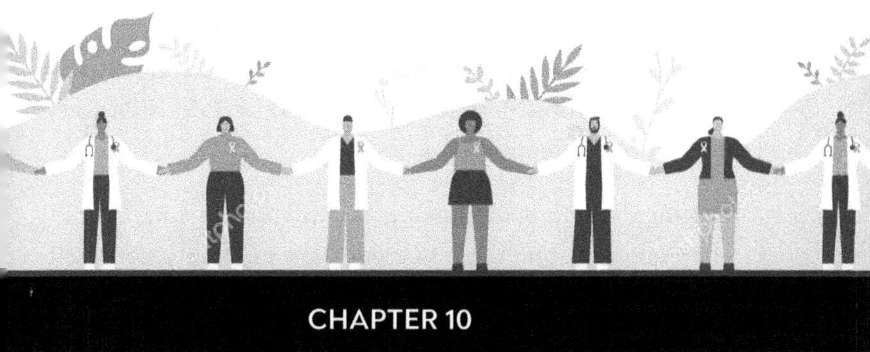

CHAPTER 10

CONCLUSION

You may have begun your journey with cancer as Adam did in *50/50*, but the tools in this book have now prepared you to plan the best treatment management you can. Understanding your cancer and the procedures involved in arriving at a diagnosis and a treatment plan allows you to have a seat at the table in discussions with your doctor and your health care team. In fact, yours is the most important seat at the table! You know what is best for you, and having input in the process will help you feel more in control.

Cancer is a complicated disease, and misdiagnosis is frequent. There are often multiple effective ways of treating your cancer, which means that you will face challenging decisions along your cancer journey. Get as much information as you can on your specific disease, get the best people around the table, and challenge the thoughts of people in your team as much as you can. You will get to the right decision—and, most importantly, that will be a decision with which you are comfortable.

Facing difficult decisions at a stressful time in your life can be daunting, but these decisions are essential. They will have a huge bearing on your quality of life in the immediate and distant future. At later points in your journey, you may face fatigue and other challenges, and you will need to lean back on the research and preparation you put in at the start. Have a decision plan in place that you can work through. Most of the process just involves getting the information you need, and once you're fully informed, you can think about what is most important to you.

Your doctor is your ally in this process: listen to them carefully and record your conversations. Do your research about what they are saying. Challenge it. Ensure you get the best and most appropriate tests. Record what you learn along the way in case you have to revisit the decision later, either because of new information or because the tumor has come back.

Wherever you are on your cancer journey, start today. Get all of your reports, scans, and doctor's notes, and read through them. Arrange an appointment with your health care team to discuss them. Look into getting a second opinion with the best and most experienced doctor for your specific cancer. You may be the patient whose tumor has a rare mutation with an excellent treatment option, such as that for an NTRK fusion, opening up a much better treatment avenue.

The most incredible stress associated with a cancer diagnosis is the unknown: a new language, new people, and new procedures. Combat the stress by arming yourself with knowledge! Once you understand why you are having a procedure and what will happen to the tissue collected, you will feel better. And once you are confident you are making the right decisions, you will feel better.

Confidence in the team you are working with will make it easier to put yourself in their hands when you need to. New challenges will inevitably emerge once you have arrived at your decision, but knowing you made the right one will prepare you to step up to them. Good luck on your journey.

HELPFUL ORGANIZATIONS & USEFUL LINKS

List of approved cancer centers:
nccn.org/home/member-institutions

National Comprehensive Cancer Network guidelines:
nccn.org/guidelines/category_1

Where to find a Comprehensive Cancer Center for a second opinion:
cancer.gov/research/infrastructure/cancer-centers/find

Databases for scientific publications:
scholar.google.com
pubmed.ncbi.nlm.nih.gov

Look up a doctor's qualifications:
docinfo.org

CANCER CHARITIES AND SUPPORT GROUPS

The Breast Cancer Research Foundation:
bcrf.org

Cancer Research Institute:
cancerresearch.org

Stand Up To Cancer:
https://standuptocancer.org/

Leukemia and Lymphoma Society:
lls.org

Ovarian Cancer Research Alliance:
ocrahope.org

Pancreatic Cancer Action Network:
pancan.org

Prevent Cancer Foundation:
preventcancer.org

Prostate Cancer Foundation:
pcf.org

Lung Cancer Research Foundation:
lungcancerresearchfoundation.org

National Brain Tumor Society:
braintumor.org

Kidney Cancer Association:
kidneycancer.org

SOURCES FOR FINDING APPROVED PHYSICIANS

The American Society of Clinical Oncology:
asco.org

The American Board of Medical Specialties:
abms.org

The American Medical Association:
ama-assn.org

The American College of Surgeons:
facs.org

Searchable database of doctors who accept Medicare:
medicare.gov

CLINICAL TRIALS

Clinicaltrials.gov:
clinicaltrials.gov

European Clinical Trials information:
ema.europa.eu

US Food and Drug Administration:
fda.gov

Office for Human Research Protections:
hhs.gov/ohrp/index.html

CONNECTING WITH LOVED ONES

Caring Bridge:
caringbridge.org

Lotsa Helping Hands:
lotsahelpinghands.com

TESTING CENTERS

Foundation Medicine:
foundationmedicine.com

Guardant Health:
guardanthealth.com

Caris Life Sciences:
carislifesciences.com

GLOSSARY & CANCER TERMINOLOGY

apoptosis: Cell death occurring as a normal and controlled mechanism of an organism's growth or development.

benign (tumor): A tumor that is not harmful due to its slow growth and noninvasive behavior.

biopsy: Removal of tissue from a part of the body for examination to determine the characteristics of a disease.

complete remission: A state in which all signs and symptoms of cancer have disappeared. Cancer is undetectable.

disease-free survival: The length of time after treatment during which no further sign of cancer is found.

DNA: Deoxyribonucleic acid, the molecule that contains the genetic code that is the blueprint for our cells and organs. It is present within all cells of all organisms.

endoscopy: A nonsurgical procedure used to examine the digestive tract. A flexible tube with a camera (endoscope) is passed down the esophagus.

epithelial cell: A cell that lines the surfaces of the body, including the skin, organs, and blood vessels.

false negative: A test result falsely indicating that a person does not have a specific disease or condition when, in fact, the person does.

false positive: A test result falsely indicating that a person has a specific disease or condition when, in fact, the person does not.

general anesthetic: The medication that puts you to sleep before you have surgery so you won't feel any pain.

germline: The genetic makeup that continues through successive generations.

grade: Describes how normal or abnormal tumor cells look under the microscope. Not to be confused with *stage* (see below).

immunohistochemistry (IHC): A laboratory method that uses antibodies to check for certain antigens (markers) in a sample of tissue.

ionizing radiation: A type of energy that ionizes atoms or molecules by removing electrons. This type of radiation is used in x-rays and CT scans.

liquid biopsy: Removal of a liquid (e.g., blood or urine) from a part of the body for examination to determine the characteristics of a disease.

lymph: A colorless fluid containing white blood cells that infiltrates the tissues and drains into the bloodstream.

lymphatic system: The vessel network by which the lymph drains into the blood from the tissues.

malignant (tumor): A tumor that is cancerous, or growing in a way that causes invasion of the surrounding tissues.

margin: The edge or border of cancer tissue that is removed during surgery.

metastasis: Development of a secondary malignant growth distant from the primary site of cancer.

microenvironment: The ecosystem that surrounds tumor cells. It includes the extracellular matrix, blood vessels, and other cells.

mutation: A change in the DNA sequence of a cell.

overall survival: The statistical length of time a patient remains alive from the date of diagnosis or the start of treatment.

personalized medicine: Uses a person's genetic and pathological profile to guide clinical decisions.

primary (tumor): The tumor at the site where the cancer originated.

prognosis: A forecast of the likely course of a disease.

progression-free survival: The percentage of people who have no tumor growth or cancer spread during or after treatment.

punch biopsy: A procedure where a small, round piece of tissue (2–12 mm) is removed using a sharp, hollow, circular instrument.

recurrence: When cancer is found again following a period of time when it could not be detected.

relapse: Deterioration after a period of improvement. For cancer, this is usually when the cancer has come back after some time.

replication: Copying or reproducing something (e.g., cells producing new identical cells or DNA making an identical copy of itself).

resection: Surgery to move all or part of a tumor.

RNA: Ribonucleic acid, the messenger molecule carrying instructions from DNA to create proteins in humans.

secondary (tumor): A tumor that has arisen at a different place in the body from the primary tumor.

sensitivity: The ability of a test to produce a positive result in an individual who has the disease.

signaling cascade: A series of chemical reactions that occur within a cell in response to a stimulus.

somatic mutation: A genetic alteration that occurs after conception; that is, one acquired during life (e.g., a genetic alteration in a tumor cell that does not affect normal cells).

specificity: The ability of a test to produce a negative result in an individual who does not have the disease.

squamous cells: Thin, flat cells which are part of the epithelium that lines the surfaces of the body.

stage: How much cancer is present in the body and where it is located. Not to be confused with *grade* (see above).

standard of care: The recommended medications for the type, grade, and stage of cancer at a certain point in a patient's course of disease.

BIBLIOGRAPHY & FURTHER READING

(in order of appearance in the text)

CHAPTER 1

Tokumo M, Toyooka S, Kiura K et al. The relationship between epidermal growth factor receptor mutations and clinicopathologic features in non-small cell lung cancers. Clin Cancer Res. 2005 Feb 1;11(3):1167-73. PMID: 15709185.

- Original report of EGFR mutations in lung cancer

Lynch TJ, Bell DW, Sordella R et al. Activating mutations in the epidermal growth factor receptor underlying responsiveness of non-small-cell lung cancer to gefitinib. N Engl J Med. 2004 May 20;350(21):2129-39. doi: 10.1056/NEJMoa040938.

- Association of EGFR mutations with response to EGFR inhibitors

Kazandjian D, Blumenthal GM, Yuan W, He K, Keegan P, Pazdur R. FDA approval of gefitinib for the treatment of patients with metastatic EGFR mutation-positive non-small cell lung cancer. Clin Cancer Res. 2016 Mar 15;22(6):1307-12. doi: 10.1158/1078-0432.CCR-15-2266.

- FDA approval of EGFR inhibitors for patients with lung cancer with EGFR mutations

Wempe MM, Stewart MD, Glass D et al. A national assessment of diagnostic test use for patients with advanced NSCLC and factors influencing physician decision-making. Am Health Drug Benefits. 2020 Jun;13(3):110-119. PMID: 32699571.

- 2020 survey of health professionals about molecular testing

McKinney SM, Sieniek M, Godbole V et al. International evaluation of an AI system for breast cancer screening. Nature. 2020 Jan;577(7788):89-94. doi: 10.1038/s41586-019-1799-6.

- Google DeepMind computer diagnosis comparison to human diagnosis

Van Such M, Lohr R, Beckman T, Naessens JM. Extent of diagnostic agreement among medical referrals. J Eval Clin Pract. 2017 Aug;23(4):870-874. doi: 10.1111/jep.12747.

- Mayo clinic study showing differences in referral diagnosis and final diagnosis

CHAPTER 2

The International Histological Classification of Tumours. Bulletin of the World Health Organization, 59 (6): 813-819 (1981).

- The first WHO book categorizing tumors based

on their original primary location, defined by histopathology

Skin cancer is the most common form of cancer in the United States. CDC. https://www.cdc.gov/cancer/skin/statistics/index.htm. Accessed April 2021.

Travis WD, Brambilla E, Burke AP, Marx A, Nicholson AN, editors. WHO classification of tumours of the lung, pleura, thymus and heart. Geneva: WHO Press; 2015.

CHAPTER 4

NCCN guidelines for soft tissue sarcoma, thyroid carcinoma, lung cancer, gastric cancer. https://www.nccn.org/guidelines/

- Treatments of tumors with NTRK fusions with an NTRK inhibitor

https://www.rozlytrek.com/content/dam/gene/rozlytrek/hcp/resources-downloads-component/pdfs/rozlytrek-nccn-flashcards-digital-pdf.pi.pdf?nocache=true

- Drug label for entrectinib (an NTRK inhibitor)

Wempe MM, Stewart MD, Glass D et al. A national assessment of diagnostic test use for patients with advanced NSCLC and factors influencing physician decision-making. Am Health Drug Benefits. 2020 Jun;13(3):110-119. PMID: 32699571; PMCID: PMC7370822.

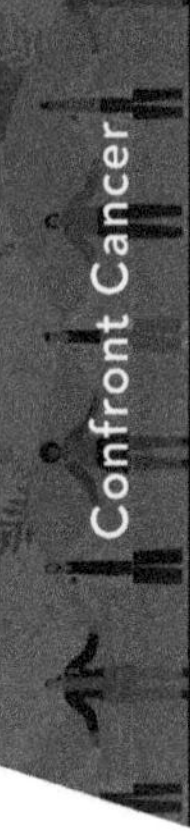

- 2019 survey of physicians managing patients with non-small cell lung cancer showing that insurance coverage affects what options a doctor presents to a patient

CHAPTER 5

Smeltzer MP, Wynes MW, Lantuejoul S et al. The International Association for the Study of Lung Cancer global survey on molecular testing in lung cancer. J Thorac Oncol. 2020 Sep;15(9):1434-1448. doi: 10.1016/j.jtho.2020.05.002. Epub 2020 May 20. PMID: 32445813.

- In this 2020 survey, only one in four doctors knew about updated policies

Baselga J, Norton L, Albanell J, Kim YM, Mendelsohn J. Recombinant humanized anti-HER2 antibody (Herceptin) enhances the antitumor activity of paclitaxel and doxorubicin against HER2/neu overexpressing human breast cancer xenografts. Cancer Res. 1998 Jul 1;58(13):2825-31. Erratum in: Cancer Res 1999 Apr 15;59(8):2020. PMID: 9661897.

- Trastuzumab for breast cancer: initial reports of activity

https://www.drugs.com/history/avastin.html Accessed April 2021.

- FDA approval history for bevacizumab (brand name Avastin)

https://www.drugs.com/history/venclexta.html Accessed April 2021.

- FDA approval history for venetoclax (brand name Venclexta)

CHAPTER 6

Jordan VC, Koerner S. Tamoxifen (ICI 46,474) and the human carcinoma 8S oestrogen receptor. Eur J Cancer. 1975 Mar;11(3):205-6. doi: 10.1016/0014-2964(75)90119-x.

- Report of tamoxifen in the 1970s

Nowell PC, Hungerford DA. Chromosome studies on normal and leukemic human leukocytes. J Natl Cancer Inst. 1960 Jul;25:85-109. PMID: 14427847.

- First association of the BCR/ABL gene fusion (also known as the Philadelphia chromosome) being associated with cancer

Kosaka T, Yatabe Y, Endoh H et al. Analysis of epidermal growth factor receptor gene mutation in patients with non-small cell lung cancer and acquired resistance to gefitinib. Clin Cancer Res. 2006 Oct 1;12(19):5764-9. doi: 10.1158/1078-0432.CCR-06-0714

- EGFR T790M mutations associated with resistance to gefitinib

CHAPTER 7

National Comprehensive Cancer Network (NCCN) guidelines. https://www.nccn.org/guidelines/

National Institute for Health and Care Excellence guidelines

https://www.nice.org.uk/about/what-we-do/our-programmes/nice-guidance/nice-guidelines

CHAPTER 8

Gierman HJ, Goldfarb S, Labrador M et al. Genomic testing and treatment landscape in patients with advanced non-small cell lung cancer (aNSCLC) using real-world data from community oncology practices. J Clin Oncol. 2019; 37(15_suppl):1585. doi: 10.1200/JCO.2019.37.15_suppl.1585.

- A majority of patients with lung cancer are only tested for mutations in the three genes most commonly found in lung cancer

Gandhi L, Rodríguez-Abreu D, Gadgeel S et al.; KEYNOTE-189 investigators. Pembrolizumab plus chemotherapy in metastatic non-small-cell lung cancer. N Engl J Med. 2018 May 31;378(22):2078-2092. doi: 10.1056/NEJMoa1801005.

- Chemotherapy and immunotherapy for NSCLC show a median survival of around 8.8 months

www.ingramcontent.com/pod-product-compliance
Ingram Content Group UK Ltd.
Pitfield, Milton Keynes, MK11 3LW, UK
UKHW020338310726
14060UKWH00020B/746/J